The Ethical Visions of Psychotherapy

Kevin R. Smith

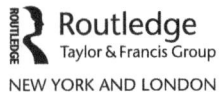

Routledge
Taylor & Francis Group

NEW YORK AND LONDON

First published 2021
by Routledge
52 Vanderbilt Avenue, New York, NY 10017

and by Routledge
2 Park Square, Milton Park, Abingdon, Oxon OX14 4RN

Routledge is an imprint of the Taylor & Francis Group, an informa business

British Library Cataloguing-in-Publication Data
A catalogue record for this book is available from the British Library

Library of Congress Cataloging-in-Publication Data
Names: Smith, Kevin R., 1953- author.
Title: The ethical visions of psychotherapy/Kevin R. Smith.
Description: New York: Routledge, 2020. |
Series: Advances in theoretical and philosophical psychology |
Includes bibliographical references and index.
Identifiers: LCCN 2020011009 (print) | LCCN 2020011010 (ebook) |
ISBN 9780367480301 (hardback) | ISBN 9780367524951 (paperback) |
ISBN 9781003039143 (ebook)
Subjects: LCSH: Psychotherapy–Moral and ethical aspects.
Classification: LCC RC455.2.E8 S63 2020 (print) |
LCC RC455.2.E8 (ebook) | DDC 616.89/14–dc23
LC record available at https://lccn.loc.gov/2020011009
LC ebook record available at https://lccn.loc.gov/2020011010

ISBN: 978-0-367-48030-1 (hbk)
ISBN: 978-1-003-03914-3 (ebk)

Typeset in Times New Roman
by Deanta Global Publishing Services, Chennai, India

For Beth, with love and gratitude

Contents

Acknowledgments

Many people and institutions have provided direct and indirect support for this work. My philosophical thinking about therapy was initially formed in my graduate training at Duquesne University. My understanding of therapy as a practitioner has been shaped by many supervisors, colleagues, supervisees, and patients over the years, as well as my own experience of being a patient in humanistic, psychoanalytic, and Jungian therapy. At the Western Psychiatric Institute and Clinic in Pittsburgh, I had the good fortune to be introduced to therapy research through my work as a therapist in multisite studies examining the efficacy of cognitive-behavioral and psychodynamic therapies. Paul Pilkonis modeled how therapy researchers can be appreciative of the depth and complexity of therapeutic process while trying to formulate well-defined research questions. Both the Pittsburgh Psychoanalytic Institute and the seminars of the "Keeping Our Work Alive" group in Pittsburgh organized by Bill Cornell have been crucial to the deepening of my understanding and practice of therapy. Brent Slife has offered much needed encouragement. I benefited from the opportunity to present an early version of portions of Chapters 3 and 4 at the 2019 Midwinter Meeting of Division 24 of the American Psychological Association (Division of Theoretical and Philosophical Psychology).

Many people have been kind enough to read and comment on portions of this work: Donna Coufal, Miriam Deriso, Louella Diaz, Derek Hook, Sharon Leak, and Ed Novak. I am particularly indebted to four people who have given extensively of their time, reading all (or most) of the book: Beth Knapp, Mark Kroll-Fratoni, Jane Matz, and Jeff McCurry. They have corrected numerous errors and made important recommendations regarding the substance and style of the argument. I am deeply grateful for their advice and support.

Series Foreword
Brent D. Slife, Editor

Psychologists need to face the facts. Their commitment to empiricism for answering disciplinary questions does not prevent pivotal questions from arising that cannot be evaluated exclusively through empirical methods, hence the title of this series: *Advances in Theoretical and Philosophical Psychology*. Such moral questions as, "What is the nature of a good life?" are crucial to psychotherapists but are not answerable through empirical methods alone. And what of the methods themselves? Many have worried that our current psychological means of investigation are not adequate for fully understanding the person (e.g., Schiff, 2019). How do we address this concern through empirical methods without running headlong into the dilemma of methods investigating themselves? Such questions are in some sense philosophical, to be sure, but the discipline of psychology cannot advance even its own empirical agenda without addressing questions like these in defensible ways.

How then should the discipline of psychology deal with such distinctly theoretical questions? We could leave the answers exclusively to professional philosophers, but this option would mean that the conceptual foundations of the discipline, including the conceptual framework of empiricism itself, are left to scholars who are *outside* the discipline. As undoubtedly helpful as philosophers are and would be, this situation would mean that the people doing the actual psychological work, psychologists themselves, are divorced from the people who formulate and re-formulate the conceptual foundations of that work. This division of labor would not seem to serve the long-term viability of the discipline.

Instead, the founders of psychology—thinkers such as Wundt, Freud, and James—recognized the importance of psychologists in formulating their own foundations. These parents of psychology not only did their own theorizing, in cooperation with many other disciplines; they realized the significance of psychologists continuously *re*-examining these theories and philosophies. This re-examination process allowed for the people most directly involved in and knowledgeable about the discipline to be the ones to decide *whether* changes were needed and *how* such changes would best be implemented. This book series is dedicated to that task, the examining and re-examining of psychology's foundations.

1 Introduction

The Means and Ends of Therapy

A central component of many of the psychotherapies is the exploration of aspects of psychological functioning that patients are initially unaware of or disavow. For example, psychoanalysis aims to bring to light wishes, motives, and aspects of the self that have been repressed or dissociated. Cognitive therapy aims to help patients see how, unbeknown to them, their thinking generates their depressed mood or anxiety.

A central aim of this book is to point to something therapists do that they don't readily acknowledge, or are even motivated to avoid. Therapists think of themselves as offering treatments for psychiatric disorders, methods to change problematic behaviors and alleviate emotional distress, or ways to improve social and work functioning. This view of therapy as a means to bring about particular ends is not false, but it is incomplete. Therapy is also a social practice that enacts some perspective on what constitutes a good life, human well-being, or flourishing. To the extent that this latter characterization of therapy is true, psychotherapy is not simply a means to an end but proposes that some ends are more worth pursuing than others. In Robinson's (1997) words, therapy "is and must be a theory about the good life; a theory about realistic and worthy pursuits; a theory about persons" (p. 676).

To think about therapy as proposing ideas about what constitutes a good life raises a number of important issues. Does such a picture of therapy apply to all therapies, even those that were expressly developed to be technical means to achieve specific ends? How can this view be reconciled with the position of many therapists who adamantly oppose telling patients how to live their lives? When a therapy seems to offer a notion of human flourishing, does this make it more than therapy, something like a philosophy of life? If ideas about what makes life worthwhile are at least implicitly present in the psychotherapies, is this a problem to be addressed, or an inevitable feature that needs to be acknowledged? And what do we do about clashes between competing pictures of human well-being that are present in different therapies? There are established methods for assessing differential therapeutic efficacy when therapy is understood as a means to a circumscribed end (as a treatment for depression or panic disorder, for example). How do we assess different ideas about human well-being?

To anticipate some of my conclusions, I will not be arguing that therapists need to develop a fully articulated theory of the good life. But I will be arguing that it is incumbent upon therapists to reflect on their implicit assumptions about what constitutes human flourishing. It is dishonest for therapists to claim that they have no ethical agendas. Therapists' attachments to broad therapeutic orientations (psychodynamic, cognitive-behavioral, humanistic, mindfulness-based, etc.) are rooted in the sense that their preferred approach provides something worthwhile that goes beyond symptom reduction. The rational self-mastery of cognitive-behavioral therapy, the search for authenticity of humanistic therapy, and the honest acknowledgment and working through of previously repressed wishes and motives in psychodynamic therapy are all offered as key components of living well.

Unreflective commitment to the picture of flourishing in one's preferred therapeutic orientation has its risks. Blind adherence can conceal the limitations of an orientation and the value of alternative approaches. But this danger is not resolved by claiming neutrality. To ignore broad ethical aims and focus only on narrowly framed questions of efficacy also has its cost, namely, that our understanding of therapy is distorted through the failure to take into account the visions of well-being implicit in therapeutic practices.

What follows is an effort to spell out the idea that the therapies include at least implicit proposals regarding what constitutes living well (an "ethic"), and that part of what is at stake between different therapies are the differences between these proposals. In Chapter 2 I articulate the link between therapeutic aims and conceptions of well-being, clarify terminology ("flourishing," "well-being," and "ethics"), and offer a preliminary justification for examining therapy in these terms. Chapters 3 and 4 provide illustrations of the link between therapy and ethics. Chapter 3 starts by exploring the idea that therapeutic efforts to improve well-being are simply attempts to restore psychological health, and as such have little to do with what we ordinarily think of as ethics. In response I examine how psychological problems implicate ideas about living well that go beyond ordinary conceptions of health. I illustrate this by examining how even therapies that were designed to target circumscribed mental disorders include broad ethical aims. In Chapter 4 I look at three different versions of psychoanalysis to show how closely related forms of therapy can be distinguished by their different ethics. Chapter 5 takes up a "So what?" question about the link between therapy and ethics: Why bother with the competing pictures of well-being in the therapies if we can simply research which therapies work better? I argue that psychotherapy research highlights the significance of the ethical disputes between the therapies, for they are generally equivalent in efficacy. I conclude with some reflections on the need to supplement the standard assessment of therapeutic efficacy with consideration of the contrasting ethical aims of different therapies. Deeper engagement in the latter task requires a better grasp of the cultural roots of therapeutic ethics and the development of a discourse of ethical evaluation and dialogue that is often missing in the field. These topics are taken up in more detail in the companion volume, *Therapeutic Ethics in Context and in Dialogue.*

Explorations of the intersection of ethics and psychotherapy do not figure centrally in dominant conceptions of therapy. To work on these topics is to labor in a peripheral corner of the field in this era of practice guidelines and evidence-based treatment. I owe a large debt to many who have already written on these topics: Atwood and Stolorow (1993), Cushman (1995, 2019), Fancher (1995), Fowers et al. (2017), Lear (2003, 2017), London (1986), Martin (2006), Miller (2004), Orange (2011), Richardson et al. (1999), Richardson and Zeddies (2004), Robinson, D. N. (1997), Stern (2012), Tjeltveit (1999), and Woolfolk (1998, 2015). They have shaped my own thinking and have provided ample evidence in their work that psychotherapy has a great deal to do with ethics.

However, my approach does not consist of a close engagement with these writers, examining points of agreement and disagreement among them, or considering how their thinking aligns with or diverges from my own views. Instead, the central thread that runs through this book is the philosophy of Charles Taylor. A key aim of his work has been to show how the evaluative and interpretive nature of human existence limits the prospects for an objectivist science of people. I rely heavily upon several themes from Taylor's work that elaborate on this central idea: the concept of strong evaluation and the inevitability of ethics; the obscuring of ethics by modern objectivist and scientistic thinking; the constitutive role of language in giving shape to our ethical views; and the holistic nature of the meanings by which we live—which is related to the holistic nature of the language through which they take form. In *Therapeutic Ethics in Context and in Dialogue* I also borrow heavily from Taylor's work on the culture of modernity in order to provide a context for therapeutic ethics and apply his ideas about practical reasoning to the prospects for dialogue between conflicting therapeutic views of flourishing. Taylor's ideas provide the anchor points and structure for the claims I want to make about therapy. Taylor does not write in detail about psychotherapy. Rather than build upon his few comments on the subject, I make use of fundamental concepts from Taylor's philosophy to develop better ways to frame some basic questions about the nature of therapy. When I enlist a major theme of his work I will give an overview of it and illustrate how it applies to the specific issue I am exploring. A background in his philosophy is not necessary to follow my argument. Those who are unfamiliar with Taylor's work and would like a summary will find a brief introduction in the appendix to *Therapeutic Ethics in Context and in Dialogue.*

2   The Ethics of Therapeutic Aims

Prologue: A Tale of Two Therapies

Jane[1] has been having panic attacks. At least she thinks they are panic attacks. That's what the doctor told her at the emergency room last week. Despite the doctor's reassurances, she's not entirely sure. She still wonders if the chest pressure, racing heart, and shortness of breath might be an indication that there is something medically wrong, and if the next time this happens she will have a heart attack, not a panic attack. The emergency room staff suggested she try therapy and gave her the names of a couple of psychotherapists.

Depending on which therapist she sees, Jane may have very different experiences. Suppose she sees Dr. Adams. Dr. Adams begins with a careful assessment, asking about the nature, intensity, and timing of Jane's symptoms; the history of their onset; the impact of these symptoms on Jane's functioning; and some general questions about Jane's life apart from this presenting problem. Seeing no other obvious difficulties that would complicate the clinical picture, Dr. Adams begins in the first few sessions to outline a formulation of the problem and to sketch a course of treatment. A summary of what she tells Jane goes something like this:

> I'm glad that the hospital ruled out any cardiac involvement, but I realize that that hasn't entirely reassured you. It can be difficult to believe that a panic attack isn't something medically serious. Part of what makes panic attacks so frightening is the belief that they are something serious. If I thought I was having a heart attack, I'd be scared too. During a panic attack the fight-or-flight response, your body's alarm system, has been triggered even though there is no real danger. It is physically intense, your heart races, you get short of breath, but it isn't dangerous. What makes it really terrible is that you think it might be something truly catastrophic. What we need to do is help you to get greater confidence that these symptoms aren't dangerous. But you'll need more than

information, more than me simply telling you they aren't dangerous. I want to work with you on ways you can be more convinced of this, through some education about panic, but more importantly, by teaching you some ways to test out your fears in order to see for yourself that you aren't in danger. This will involve learning a method to carefully think through your fears and some practical exercises that will help you train yourself not to react automatically with fear to these bodily sensations.

If Jane goes to see Dr. Bonn things may start in a similar fashion. Dr. Bonn will ask about what Jane is looking for help with and listen carefully to Jane's descriptions of her symptoms, sometimes asking for further details about the context in which the panic attacks arise and what Jane fears about them. Dr. Bonn, however, is more interested than Dr. Adams in the details of Jane's life circumstances apart from her panic attacks. He is not just interested in ruling out co-morbid diagnoses, but wants to know the broader concerns of Jane's life, her relationships, her work and family life, etc. A fair amount of the preliminary sessions are spent on exploring Jane's personal history, including other times in her life that have been difficult for her, what she is currently happy about and frustrated with in her life, and at least some inquiry into her childhood. Dr. Bonn will be listening not just to what Jane says, but also to how she says it. Is her self-description impressionistic, angry, or filled with extraneous details? And how does Jane seem to be positioning herself toward Dr. Bonn? As an unworthy and helpless supplicant? As a stoic sufferer who doesn't really need help? Over the course of these early sessions Dr. Bonn begins to formulate a picture of what may be amiss for Jane beyond her panic attacks. In contrast with Dr. Adams, Dr. Bonn places less emphasis on the therapeutic role of providing Jane with information about her symptoms. He is likely to offer early reflections in a less definitive way, and the following message may be given piecemeal in short comments across several meetings, rather than as an overall summary.

I can hear how frightening these panic attacks are for you and that you're eager for them to stop. I also hear there are a number of other problems that have been overwhelming, and that you feel helpless to change. You spoke of feeling trapped in your job and angry with your husband for his lack of effort in helping you with the kids and the household chores. But you also say that you're afraid to confront him, afraid that he'll leave you, which might only make everything even more impossible to manage. You said that feeling trapped like this also reminds you of your mother's situation when you were growing up. You were determined not to repeat her mistakes and now you sound despondent, even embarrassed, that you may be in a similar position. Your panic attacks have something to do with feeling backed into a corner in your life. I think that addressing your panic will require doing something about these binds that keep you from living the kind of life you would like to live.

Both Dr. Adams and Dr. Bonn conclude their initial assessment sessions and feedback with an inquiry as to whether their respective preliminary understandings and suggestions about how to proceed make sense to Jane. In both cases the therapists are inviting Jane to make an initial endorsement of a particular take on human psychology and of how to understand problems like hers in light of their approach. Dr. Adams paints a picture of persons as psychological systems shaped by biology, conditioning, and cognition, systems which can be re-worked to ameliorate symptoms like her recurring panic attacks. Dr. Bonn focuses on the patient's frustrations with her job and marriage, what makes her feel helpless to change things, as well as her concern that she has failed to be the kind of person she has aspired to be. Each of these therapists is proposing a different way of relating to oneself and of addressing difficulties in living. Each is emphasizing different ideas about the most important elements of being human. One might object that these ideas about how to understand people are brought to bear upon the specific problem of panic disorder. They are not offered as a general psychology or as an approach for handling all aspects of life. But this way of putting the matter is not innocent. For to suggest that the heart of the matter is treatment of panic disorder as a free-standing problem is already to lean toward one way of understanding human difficulties. It is to begin to side with Dr. Adams over Dr. Bonn.

Different therapies are rooted in different takes on what it is to be human, how problems in living arise, what makes something a problem, and how to go about making things better. In short, different therapies rely on different philosophical anthropologies, although they are rarely discussed in such terms by therapists and researchers. Instead, the arguments are often framed in terms of questions about whether one therapy is more effective than another at treating the symptoms of a disorder, or whether one delves more deeply into the psychological roots of various problems. One consequence of avoiding the more fundamental questions of philosophical anthropology is that the opposing sides in these arguments often talk past each other. I want to offer some suggestions about how to deepen these debates by offering a different way to think about what is at stake.

Therapy Wars

Current views of psychotherapy often seem to issue from camps that battle one another blindly. The camps are sometimes divided based on therapeutic orientation. Cognitive-behaviorists, humanists, and psychodynamic therapists tout the merits of their respective therapies and focus on flaws of the other therapies, flaws that seem obvious when viewed through the lens of their own approach. Warring camps are also formed around different ways to study therapy. Clinical experience is pitted against research and both are critiqued by those who examine therapy with the tools of social, cultural, or political analysis. The arguments are unresolved and partisans retreat to conferences, institutes, and journals where they find like-minded people.

When I say that there is a fair amount of "blind battling" in disputes about therapy, I am suggesting two things. One is that various therapies and methods for studying therapy often operate from a narrow or distorted picture of alternative views. The other is that I think there is potential value in a more robust dialogue among the contrasting positions. That dialogue can be deepened by examining an aspect of psychotherapy that I want to highlight. The one-sided nature of the positions often held in therapy debates is rooted in attachment to something more than a scientific conception of psychological disorder and what may alleviate it. The interlocutors in these debates are also often devoted to a personally and intellectually compelling conception of human well-being. Dedication to the improvement of the human condition (whether this is couched in psychological, political, or other terms) often comes in the form of passionate investments that can make competing views appear to be not just incorrect but also dangerous and harmful. For example, proponents of longer term, exploratory or psychodynamic psychotherapies indict short-term treatments that focus on symptom reduction as quick fixes for the superficial manifestations of more complex problems. The psychodynamic and humanistic therapies are critiqued in turn as exercises in endless, expensive self-exploration that fail to offer interventions that have been proven to be effective means to change crippling symptomatology. Social critics of therapy note the ways that psychotherapy can abet unjust social or economic structures. The targets of critique in each of these examples are seen as not simply wrong, but as doing damage, as obstructing some possibility for living well in just social arrangements. Yet, the role of conflicting visions of well-being in these debates is rarely productively addressed.

One can approach these arguments about therapy from markedly different perspectives and get very different answers. Therapy practitioners and theorists, psychotherapy researchers, historians, and social critics have proposed a wide variety of views on what therapy is and what aims it serves or ought to serve. These perspectives can be roughly sorted into three basic approaches: (1) the empirical-technical; (2) the promotion of values or ideals; and (3) the socio-historical.

The Empirical-Technical Perspective on Therapy

From this perspective psychotherapy is viewed as a psychological intervention intended to change a pattern of behavior or treat a mental disorder. Examples of this perspective abound in the psychotherapy literature. It is often associated with manualized behavioral and cognitive-behavioral treatments (for a survey of these treatments, see Barlow, 2014). While such treatments may be paradigmatic examples, this perspective is present in many approaches to therapy. It is at least implicitly present in any effort to develop therapy as an effective intervention for a specific problem, be that therapy short-term or long-term, cognitive-behavioral, humanistic, or psychodynamic. For example, Breuer and Freud (1893/1955) write of the disappearance of hysterical symptoms when an affectively engaged memory of the event that provoked the symptoms is put into words by the patient. Insofar as this is turned into a technique to treat hysteria, it would be an example of the empirical-technical perspective. This perspective is also at the heart of research that investigates the efficacy of psychotherapy. The picture of flourishing in this perspective is usually not explicitly articulated. It is simply the state that is restored when the behavior, symptom, or disorder that is the target of the therapy is removed. However, as I will examine in the next chapter, implicit in this view is the idea of flourishing as a capacity to direct one's own life, to be an autonomous agent.

Therapy as the Promotion of Specific Values or Ideals

From this perspective therapy is conceived as promoting a more explicitly formulated good. Understood in this light, psychotherapy does not simply remove a problem, symptom, or disorder, but sustains a particular conception of flourishing. For example, Nancy McWilliams (2005) proposes that therapy can benefit patients and society through the promotion of values of self-understanding, authenticity, empathy and compassion, egalitarianism, adaptation to unchangeable realities, growth in agency and personal responsibility, acceptance of normal dependency, and respect for others as subject rather than object. Some cognitive-behavioral therapists (Ellis, 1962; Robinson, 2010) espouse the virtue of equanimity in the face of what cannot be changed and the value of reason in living a life free of neurosis. Sometimes the picture of human flourishing is less an explicitly stated value than an ideal implied in the practice of the therapy. The cognitive therapy procedure of challenging irrational thinking points to rationality as a human good, whether or not a therapist directly offers to patients a justification for adopting rationality as essential to living well. Similarly, psychoanalytic free association is a therapeutic practice that has been viewed as implicitly supporting an ethic of honesty (Thompson, 2004).

The Socio-Historical Perspective on Therapy

Whether therapeutic enhancement of flourishing is given a relatively thin characterization as simply removing obstacles to independent agency, or is given a more specific content (self-understanding, authenticity, empathy, rationality, honesty, etc.), one can also ask about the significance of these aims and values within a particular socio-historical context. This context can help to illuminate what is appealing about the picture of well-being on offer in a therapy. Ideas about what it means to live well are not invented by individual therapists working in isolation but arise out of a cultural matrix that helps to shape those ideals. Further, social and cultural influences on ideas about living well may be so widely accepted that they are taken for granted and promoted in therapy without therapists realizing that there are alternatives. For example, Aron and Starr (2013) examine how the influence of modern Western ideals of autonomy and rationality shaped psychoanalytic thinking to over-pathologize dependency in patients and denigrate support-ive interventions. Others argue that therapists may think they are promoting one ideal, when the cultural or political context suggests they are serving other ends. For example, Foucault (1976/1978) contends that psychoanaly-sis does not so much seek to undo the harm caused by societal prohibitions against sex as to participate in the power that takes charge of and deploys sex. Cushman (1995) describes how psychotherapy has served the agendas of American capitalism.

In order to understand the role that ideas about human flourishing play in therapy, all three perspectives need to be considered. A number of problems are generated by the tendency to emphasize one perspective at the expense of the others. The univocal focus on empirical questions regarding what works in therapy can obscure the fact that the removal of impediments to "mental health" (often left undefined) can have significant ethical and social impli-cations. Questions about whether and how therapy works need to be sup-plemented by more fundamental questions about psychotherapy's aims. The problematic ethics of what are proposed as technical therapeutic aims are obvious in some cases, such as past efforts to "cure" homosexuality. But the focus on what works in therapy may lead to more subtle ethical problems. The taken-for-granted idea of a psychological problem as something internal to a self-contained psyche or organism, something to be repaired or modified by an effective intervention, can obscure the ways in which the problem and its solution are implicated in and partake of various ethical ideas and social practices. For example, decreasing the harsh self-criticism of people suffer-ing from introjective depression (Blatt, 2004) may lead them to change their standards for moral self-assessment. But then this is not just the treatment of a depressive disorder, but an intervention in ethics that aims at a better life through less exacting moral standards. This change may be applauded on psychological grounds as effective treatment. It may also be approved on ethical grounds, for moralists have long understood that excessive scrupulosity is a threat to ethical judgment. But to frame it only as effective psychological treatment for a mental disorder is to ignore at least part of what is going on here.

There are corresponding risks in overemphasizing the promotion of particular values and ideals. For example, therapeutic techniques and theories are sometimes endorsed because they protect the autonomy of patients, as though patient autonomy were a self-evident good. What is then overlooked is the way therapeutic support for autonomy may further a particular cultural aim, such as the modern Western ideal of an individual who asserts their independence from tradition, communal ties, and the power of social and political authority. Further, this ideal may be a realistic or readily available option only for those in privileged social positions. Autonomy is neither universally valued nor equally within reach but takes on a specific set of meanings and importance that can be seen only when examined in socio-cultural context.

At the same time, the therapeutic ideals cannot be supported without some attention to the empirical perspective. A cognitive-behavioral therapist may well continue to uphold the value of rationality even after research has shown that therapeutic benefit is not the result of the correction of cognitive distortions (Imber et al., 1990; Kazdin, 2007). However, if therapies that included cognitive interventions had poorer outcomes than those that did not (which happily is not the case) some revision of the role of rationality in therapy might be needed. That is, values and ideals that make up pictures of human flourishing do not exist in a self-contained sphere. Empirical findings have some role to play in generating, supporting, and critiquing such ideals, even if the latter cannot be directly derived from the former.

Neither can the socio-historical perspective provide the final word on psychotherapy. The explanation of therapeutic practices and aims in terms of economic, political, or cultural forces that engender them can deepen our understanding of them and serve an important critical function. But critique can change practice by being incorporated into it. A political critique of a social practice that clarifies where the participants' understanding of that practice is incomplete or distorted can initiate a re-examination of the practice by the practitioners. The outcome may be that the practitioners re-work or even strengthen their practice in light of the critique. For example, one can read the history of feminist critique of psychoanalysis as leading to a transformation of theory and practice that results in a richer, more robust feminist psychoanalysis (Dimen & Goldner, 2005).

Even when socio-historical, economic, and political critiques are not incorporated by therapists, they still should not be assumed to present the "real" motivations behind what therapy practitioners and theorists mistakenly believe their aims to be. Gnaulati (2018) writes about the pressures put upon therapists from health insurers to provide short-term problem-focused treatments as a way to cut costs and increase profits. Certainly these market forces have had a problematic influence on the overall landscape of therapeutic practice. Moreover, even these forces have been distorted by insurance companies, as Gnaulati points out (that is, there is evidence that it would be cost effective to provide more generous psychotherapy benefits). But it would be misleading to think that this is the root of all problem-focused therapies. Part of the impetus for the development of cognitive-behavioral therapies, for example, has been a search for briefer and more effective treatments for psychological problems. Most therapists and therapy researchers who favor short-term therapies do not do so because they wish to enhance the profits of insurance companies. I think those who take a pragmatic approach to solving delimited psychological problems are motivated by something they share with therapists who practice other types of therapy. They are enamored of a vision of better living that is carried by that therapy's theory and practice. For cognitive-behavioral therapists, this is a vision of better living through effective and empirically supported formulations of life's difficulties as solvable problems.

I think there are serious limitations to this approach, but it is motivated by more than profits (even when it serves them). There is an ideal of efficiency here that is larger than the efficiency of market forces. Careful investigation of the causes of natural phenomena in order to gain the capacity to more efficiently change or control them is part of what modern science is about. It is important not to lose sight of the role of this scientific ideal as a motivation for many therapists and researchers simply because some promoters of short-term therapy, and some insurance companies, have misused or exploited it.

However, when applied to people, this scientific ideal also has important links to broader ideas about how to live well, supporting an ethic of reflective self-mastery and effective problem-solving. These values are not obviously amenable to empirical justification, especially when contrasted with alternative pictures of human flourishing. Not everyone views all human difficulties as problems that call for effective intervention. Some therapeutic ideas about well-being might emphasize the contemplation of mystery and fate in one's life, the exploration and development of one's particular way of living, and the playful yet serious creativity necessary to embark on such endeavors.

Fundamental frameworks for living well are not easily supportable with data, much less are they self-evident. It is not a given of human nature that each of us will be interested in "the exploration and development of one's particular way of living." Both this aim and the ideal of living one's life with problem-solving efficiency have a history and location in the modern West that gives them a particular significance.[2] Any one of the therapeutic aims and their attendant pictures of human well-being may well be worthwhile, even worth fighting for. But they are not simply natural facts about people. They take on their sense, significance, and value in the context of particular socio-historical locations.

I have so far been painting a picture of opposing camps locked in battle. But not everyone who examines competing views of therapy is firmly ensconced in one perspective. Many therapists are eclectic in their practice or have attempted to systematically integrate different therapeutic orientations. Further, some who are wedded to one school of therapy are also serious researchers, or also attend to the socio-historical context of psychotherapy and of the problems it attempts to address. There are efforts to bridge the differences. But those who engage in bridging efforts have the same difficulties that the more adamant proponents of one therapeutic orientation or of one approach to the study of therapy have. Instead of questions about which therapy is better, or which perspective for explaining therapy is better, the questions are about what is gained and what is lost in the effort to bring together different therapeutic practices or ways of studying therapy. For example, are the different ways that cognitive-behavioral therapy and psychoanalysis conceptualize patient autonomy combinable? Would putting together practices and techniques from each of them water down what is most distinctive and laudatory about their respective aims? Would a hybrid or synthesized notion of autonomy represent a gain or a loss? How would we decide?

Clarifying Terminology: "Ethics"

Given the central role I am giving to terms such as "ethics," "human flourishing," "well-being," and "a good life," I would like to give some preliminary indications of what I am referring to with this language. One concept that comes close to the central meaning of these terms as I use them is Aristotle's (trans., 1984) eudaimonia (a "happiness" that is not so much feeling good as living well). These terms together point to a family of overlapping concepts having to do with the assessment of what is worthwhile in living one's life, what makes for a fulfilling or exemplary life.

Some of these terms are in fairly wide use among psychologists. "Flourishing" has recently been used in psychology (e.g., Keyes, 2007) to designate something beyond the absence of mental disorder that is essential to human well-being. Flourishing includes positive states of emotion, and of psychological and social functioning. Positive psychology (Seligman, 2011; Seligman & Csikszentmihalyi, 2000; Seligman et al., 2005) also emphasizes the positive qualities and activities that are essential to a well-lived life. Positive features of flourishing can be neglected when clinical theorists focus exclusively on the causes and cure of mental illness. This distinction between the positive features of flourishing and the absence of mental disorders is an important one. But it is not the focus of my use of the term. For one thing, I am going to examine how even therapies that are intended to correct or ameliorate mental disorders include at least implicit notions of flourishing. Further, positive psychology's view of flourishing can generate a rosy picture of being able to construct or engineer one's happiness (for a valuable corrective to this tendency, see Fowers et al., 2017). Some therapeutic views of flourishing or human well-being have this more positive aura about them. But not all. Freud is famous for his reservations about how much success people can have in their efforts to manage the conflicts between sexual drives and societal expectations. Existential psychotherapy's call to face death, existential isolation, or meaninglessness (Yalom, 1980) hardly constitutes an optimistic picture of human well-being. But pictures of well-being these darker views nonetheless are. Freud and the existentialists would argue that this is as good as it gets, and that the effort to paint over the inherently tragic aspects of life with too much positivity is likely to generate greater misery.

"Flourishing" and "well-being" can have connotations different from "living well" or "living a good life." When soldiers bravely sacrifice themselves to save their fellow soldiers their self-sacrifice may be pointed to as evidence of their having lived well. But one would not ordinarily say that their deaths constitute a form of well-being. Nevertheless, some might speak of this sacrifice as a form of flourishing, claiming that it is better to die courageously in battle for one's comrades than to live a long life that is cramped and lifeless because constricted by timidity. People can define terms such as flourishing and living well in very different ways. I am using these terms as open markers for a variety of ethical positions. Ethics lays out what constitutes a good life, what makes it worthwhile, what is the best we can attain. Some ethics may claim that living a good life, human flourishing, is to be found in doing well by others, even at great cost to oneself. Other ethics do not focus on the good of others as the point of life. For example, Thompson (2004) contends that psychoanalytic free association implicitly promotes an ethic of honesty. He argues that the fundamental aim of psychoanalysis is truth, in the specific sense of "disclosing what we dare about ourselves to another" (p. xx). The implication is that whatever other outcomes may ensue for the patient (decrease in neurotic symptoms, having more energy, etc.) these benefits exist on a foundation of interpersonal honesty that takes place in the treatment. For Thompson, honesty is the central ethic embodied in psychoanalytic practice, not devoting oneself to the good of others.

Is it legitimate to lump together under the heading of ethics both those ideas that define living well in terms of our fundamental moral obligations to each other, and those that define living well in terms of material, social, or psychological goods that individuals may seek for their own benefit? At first glance, the two seem to point to distinctly different concepts, even if one can imagine an overarching framework that combines them. There have been many philosophical efforts to spell out the essence of our obligations to others. Kant (1785/1997) sees the essence of moral action to lie not in inclination or desire (not even in a desire to do good for others), but in rational apprehension of and respect for the law, in understanding that the good that one would do is required by reason. Utilitarian views (Mill, 1861/1979) regarding our fundamental obligations base them on an assessment of that which would generate the greatest good, understood as the greatest pleasure, happiness, or "utility." Levinas's (1961/1969) phenomenological account attempts to describe ethics as an event in which the encounter with the other as beyond my grasp (the "face") places me in a position of infinite demand, of limitless responsibility for the other.

By contrast with these efforts to define the essence of our obligations to others, views regarding what makes a life full, complete, or worthwhile encompass a broad range of evaluative ideas and social practices. Such ethics are variable, the products of socio-cultural context. Living life well means something different to a Homeric era warrior, a medieval French monk, and a contemporary middle-class suburban American. Much of what is central to pictures of flourishing has little to do with fundamental moral obligations to others such as truthfulness or respect for others' lives, liberty, and welfare. For example, Thompson's sense of honesty ("disclosing what we dare about ourselves to another") is clearly part of a proposal about how to live life well. It is not clear that it is a moral imperative in the sense that the norm of truth telling is. Further, there are a variety of modern ideas about living well that emphasize the centrality of enjoying, expressing, or liberating oneself. These ethics have sometimes been formulated in such a way as to be opposed to any sense of obligation to others. As one Lacanian analyst puts it: "Do not act in accordance with what you believe to be the good of your fellow man or woman: act in accordance with your own desire" (Fink, 2014b, p. 57).

So it would seem that fundamental ideas regarding what we owe each other (such as those articulated in moral philosophy) are quite distinct from ethical ideas about what constitutes a flourishing life. However, while one can distinguish them conceptually, Charles Taylor argues that in practice they are interwoven (see Taylor, 2016, pp. 201–204; 1989, chapter 3). He points to three ways in which they are bound to each other. First, in applying and interpreting fundamental moral obligations we often rely on ideas about what is essential to a full, well-lived life. He takes as an example the fundamental moral principle that one ought not to infringe upon the liberty of others. There are trivial and substantive infringements upon liberty. A seat belt law infringes upon one's freedom to drive without wearing a seatbelt. But this infringement of liberty is not comparable to restrictions on free speech, the right to assembly, or the exercise of religion. Our notion of a full, flourishing life includes the value of developing and expressing one's views, being able to share them with others, or celebrating with others one's most deeply held sense of what makes life meaningful (whether this sense is religious or not). The right to drive without a seat belt is not integral to more deeply held views of a worthwhile life. The libertarian who would dispute such a law is fighting against state intrusion into citizens' lives, not for a "right" to drive free of seat belts that is equivalent to a right to free speech. "Interpreting the scope of the liberty to be respected requires us to take account of what is really important in human life, which is a key to ethics, that is, to any conception of the good life" (Taylor, 2016, p. 201).

One can raise similar issues in the context of psychotherapy. Whether therapists subscribe to Kantian or utilitarian foundations for their ethics, their therapeutic actions will involve specific choices in specific contexts that reflect assumptions about flourishing that give a particular shape to their understanding about what constitutes their duty or enhances the patient's happiness. For example, humanistic therapists who are relatively comfortable answering patients' questions about some aspects of their lives believe they owe their patients genuineness. Classical analysts who do not answer such questions may believe their obligations to their patients require maintaining an anonymous stance that allows the development and analysis of a transference neurosis. Therapists of either school may claim to be acting in the spirit of any of the more fundamental philosophical analyses of our obligations to others.

The Levinasian call to recognize our infinite responsibility to the other requires that we avoid any "totalizing" effort to subsume a patient within a particular therapeutic theory. But this requirement applies to every therapeutic orientation and will not help to assess the relative worth of different therapeutic pictures of flourishing. It is not clear that one should (or could) do therapy without any sense of what makes a life worthwhile, with no conception of flourishing. In the fundamental Levinasian ethical encounter the therapist's ideas about a good life recede into the background. But in therapeutic practice there will also be an effort to assist the patient to move from a problematic position to a better one. Notions of what is better, of what constitutes well-being, will be involved, even if they are changed in the course of therapy.

A second way in which fundamental obligations to others and ideas about human flourishing are joined comes from the fact that we are charged by fundamental moral principles with the duty to carry them out. To be able to do so can require abilities or skills that then become identified with a good life. For example, we can come to admire someone for always treating others fairly and with respect. To enact moral principles of fairness and respect becomes part of what leads us to assess someone's life as a good one, as admirable or worthwhile. The principle may appear formal, to be at the very core of what we owe to others. But enacting it becomes characteristic of a full and flourishing life.

Fundamental moral obligations are connected to ethics in a third sense. These principles have a history. Consider the contemporary idea that rights to life and liberty are owed to all people, regardless of whether they belong to a particular nation, gender, or racial group. This clearly has not always been the case, when what predominated in the past were more parochial ideas that "we" matter and deserve moral consideration in ways that "they" don't. Exclusionary views are still present today (and we often do as poorly in practice as our forebears). But the principle of universalism in the application of moral duties was not even conceived of at earlier stages of human history before the transformations wrought by various religious, philosophical, and political reformers (from the Axial Age to the Enlightenment and beyond). Further, we have a sense that in developing and aspiring to a more truly universal application of moral principles we are moving forward to a better world, a greater fulfillment of the best that we can aspire to, to a more complete picture of human flourishing. "But then the highest principles of morality define also an ethical ideal, a view of the good life" (Taylor, 2016, p. 203).[3]

If the psychotherapies promote views of the good life, this is clearly a version of ethics that is distinct from that of professional ethics codes. The contrast between these two conceptions of ethics is instructive. For example, consider the call for psychologists to uphold principles of beneficence and nonmaleficence, to work to benefit their patients and to do no harm (American Psychological Association, 2017). In the context of professional ethics, these abstract principles are illustrated in terms of the specific activities that constitute psychologists' services. For example, there is discussion of the need for psychologists to understand the limits of their expertise so that they do not offer help when they do not have the skills to actually benefit their patients. And there are prohibitions against behaviors that may undermine treatment or do psychological harm to patients, such as boundary violations (entering into business or sexual relationships with patients).

The ethics of the psychotherapies, their conceptions of human flourishing, provide another type of content to principles such as beneficence and nonmaleficence. The ethics of different therapies emphasize the value of particular benefits and propose to address corresponding harms. These proposals are quite specific and consequently could not be incorporated into an ethics code for the entire profession. No code of professional ethics could claim that the principle of beneficence obligates therapists to promote a rational and empirical method for pursuing one's own interests as in cognitive-behavioral therapy. Nor could a professional code require therapists to work to develop the discerning attunement to one's defensive operations that one acquires through Paul Gray's (1994) version of psychoanalysis. (I spell out these two therapeutic ethics in more detail in the next two chapters.) It is appropriate that beneficence remain abstract at the level of professional codes because professionals, and those whom professionals aim to benefit, need the option to find their way toward their own sense of what would be a better life. In fact, this is one source of the controversy surrounding efforts to prescribe the use of empirically supported treatments. The debate is partly about whether the research data justify these prescriptions. But there is also a concern that in prescribing a particular type of treatment one is prescribing an ethic, a picture of what sort of life people should aspire to.

In what follows I will be looking at the ethics implicit in the psychotherapies, at ways in which they propose pictures of human flourishing, and at some of the differences and similarities between those pictures. Sometimes the ethics embedded in a therapy will include specific proposals about what makes life good, worthwhile, or admirable (self-mastery achieved through rationality, or authenticity, or acting in accordance with one's own desire, etc.). Faced with a particular ethic, I may ask myself: Am I convinced or inspired to shape my life that way, and to offer it to patients as constitutive of flourishing? Does it seem attainable, whether it appeals to the patient or not? In what ways would it make my patient's life better, and what are its limitations, what does it leave out?

By focusing on ethics as aiming at a picture of human flourishing or well-being I am not suggesting that therapists ought to deliberately espouse explicitly articulated values the way that McWilliams or Thompson do in the passages quoted earlier. What I am suggesting is that therapists will inevitably be promoting some picture of flourishing in their therapies, whether explicitly spelled out or not. I am recommending reflection on one's implicit view of what is central to human well-being. Part of the motivation for this book is to promote such reflection. At the very least, therapists should be willing to acknowledge that their work is not simply a technology of psychological change, but engages with questions about what constitutes a good life.

Why Ethics?

I want to make a case for the value of examining psychotherapy in terms of its ethical assumptions. I think that viewing therapy from this perspective reveals something essential about it, and about what is at stake between the different psychotherapies. It will be the task of the remainder of this book to demonstrate this. But I can begin to sketch the rationale for examining the ethics of therapy in a preliminary fashion. This rationale is built upon a particular understanding of the participants in therapy, of the nature of persons. My explication of the idea that therapy has an intrinsic ethical component builds upon fundamental ideas of Charles Taylor's philosophical anthropology. Taylor argues that persons are agents for whom questions about what is genuinely important are unavoidable (see his papers, "What Is Human Agency?", "Self-Interpreting Animals," and "The Concept of a Person," in 1985a). This means that persons have concerns that go beyond those we share with our fellow animals. We share with non-human animals the fact that things matter to us. It matters to a dog or a mouse whether it has food and other necessities for survival. Its relations to its conspecifics, or in a dog's case, to its owners, also matter. The proper environment in which to exercise its capacities for movement, exploration, and play also matters.

Humans have similar concerns. We too have conditions of survival and ordinary desires for things like food, sex, freedom of movement, and play. But much of what matters for us is not given as fundamental needs that are built into us. We have a second layer of significance, one that addresses the worth or value of our goals and aims. That is, much of what matters to us is constituted through an evaluative appraisal made in the light of articulable standards. This transforms the significance of even the fundamental needs of life that we share with other animals. Those needs are lived and understood by us in relation to standards. We don't just feed; we dine. We can fail to meet standards. Unlike pigs, we can eat like pigs (pigs just eat). We don't just court and copulate. Flirting and attractiveness can be raised to an art form. Both falling in love and suffering heartache can have significance within a framework of ideals for living well. We don't just play; we play games that follow rules, rules that are the basis both for declaring a penalty and for challenging one. And these rules can be re-written.

I want to emphasize the foregoing phrase, "evaluative appraisal made in the light of articulable standards." Animals act for the benefit of others, sometimes even at their own expense. They can perceive and they react to situations of unfairness. They follow standards and even punish or ostracize conspecifics that deviate from expected social behavior.[4] Further, there is evidence that many human standards have evolutionary roots that we share with our fellow mammals. But non-human animals do not assess, critique, or revise the standards that they follow or fail to follow.[5] Not only are humans capable of "eating like pigs," they are capable of challenging this standard. "You're right. My table manners aren't very polished. But I think you overdo this to prove your status as upper class. I sometimes find it tiresome." Or the whole idea of moral standards may be globally critiqued, in a sophisticated philosophy like Nietzsche's, or in a crude, self-serving way: "Being good is a chump's game." Or we can argue for an extension or enhancement of standards: "It is not enough that we uphold human rights. We need to extend rights to non-human animals."

So if we can see some sense of fairness in our fellow animals, a sense that functions as a standard, it matters that that sense is not articulable by them. To articulate a sense of fairness is not simply to designate something that has already been identified apart from the articulation. To articulate standards is to give them a distinctive shape and significance that they acquire only in the articulation. Taylor (2016) refers to this as the constitutive function of language, as opposed to the use of language to designate objects that we know independently of our terms for them. The constitutive role of language is especially important for how people understand, live by, and change standards (ethical, aesthetic, political, etc.). Consider the following example.

> When I come for the first time to feel that one of the things which matters crucially to me is following my own path, finding my own way of being human (in other words, when I embrace an ethic of authenticity), I change the shape of what matters to me. I might feel (and people frequently do) that I have been feeling this all along, and just now am recognizing it, but this recognition gives a new force and clarity to this meaning. It is not like discovering the name of the odd breed of dog my neighbor walks every morning. The discovery has motivational force.
>
> (Taylor, 2016, pp. 190–191)

The different psychotherapies have different ways of articulating the ills that people suffer from and correspondingly different ways of picturing the better life that therapy aims to help patients achieve. When cognitive-behavioral therapists begin to address patients' panic attacks by offering an explanation in terms of the fight-or-flight response, they are also implicitly recommending a disengaged observational stance toward their problems. When a humanistic therapist responds to a patient's description of a recent panic attack, a different way of framing the nature of the problem may be on offer: "It sounds like you were completely overwhelmed, afraid you would die, and clung to your child in terror—and you feel ashamed that at that moment you were looking to your six-year-old daughter to comfort you." Rather than a distancing stance toward a powerful emotion, the humanistic therapist is offering an empathic re-immersion in the experience that begins to address the patient's shame over helpless dependence. When the behavioral therapist suggests exercises that promote physical sensations such as shortness of breath or a racing heart, sensations that occur during panic, this immersive experience has a different aim: to render the patient less likely to respond with fear in order to achieve (to quote the title of a popular book) "mastery of your anxiety and panic" (Barlow & Craske, 2007). The humanistic therapist is not pointing to mastery of panic through exposure and rational self-observation, but to compassionate self-acceptance in order to move away from the shame that is wrapped around the panic. The proximal aim of addressing panic attacks is approached in very different terms that significantly alter where the therapy is headed, what the more "distal" picture of human flourishing is.

In addition to the transformation of ordinary life needs (food, sex, play, etc.), the fact that we assess and shape our aims according to standards allows for the possibility that things can matter for us that aren't tied to basic life goals or aims, like the ethic of authenticity in the foregoing quote from Taylor. These standards are enormously varied. I may expect myself to be loyal to my family, competitive in business, courageous in battle, reverent in church. I don't just want to do these things; I feel it is right to do them. Such aims are available only for someone who takes a step back from simply wanting things to assessing whether something is right or worthwhile to want. For any sense that something is important to me, matters, or is desirable, I can always ask further questions about the worth of that thing. Is it truly important? Does it really matter? Have I misunderstood its importance? Is this even my own aim, or have I mindlessly taken on what others say is worthwhile? Taylor's (1985a) distinction between weak and strong evaluation is central here.

> In weak evaluation, for something to be judged good, it is sufficient that it be desired, whereas in strong evaluation there is also a use of "good" or some other evaluative term for which being desired is not sufficient; indeed some desires or desired consummations can be judged as bad, base, ignoble, trivial, superficial, unworthy, and so on.
>
> (p. 18)

With strong evaluation what I want is put to the test, examined, or supported by a standard against which the want is judged. This evaluation may or may not be explicitly carried out. It can be implicit in my acceptance of standards that I follow through my day-to-day embodied practices, without having explicitly articulated them. Many of the ideals of my culture I learn to embrace through the patterns of living into which I am inducted from a young age without having to think much about them. But they are standards nevertheless, and should those standards fail me, or I them, I can make a more deliberate reflection on them, perhaps re-affirming them, perhaps critiquing or abandoning them.

In proposing pictures of human flourishing, the psychotherapies are offering ideas about what matters at the level of strong evaluation. In being strong evaluators, patients' focal problems are partly shaped by their concerns about what matters, what human flourishing looks like, and how they can make their peace with the less than ideal. Different therapies offer contrasting strong evaluations. Does human flourishing come from the development of a nuanced appreciation and acceptance of the complexities of our motives and desires or from a stance of disengagement from our emotional life that allows us to observe, modify, or retrain it? What would it mean to affirm the former against the latter, or to try to combine them? Is this a factual disagreement about "how people work," or is this better understood as contrasting proposals for how to live that go beyond what can be factually established through objective psychological research?

Sometimes therapists deny that there are any issues of strong evaluation in therapy. They may claim that therapy is simply the utilization of psychological science to develop methods that change or treat specific behaviors or disorders. The idea seems to be that one can talk about human life without strong evaluation, that what matters to people is just as factual as, for example, that plants need water. Freud sometimes wrote this way, claiming that his only overarching framework for the understanding of psychological matters is that of science (Freud, 1933/1964) and that psychoanalysis was simply a report of scientific findings. Some proponents of empirically supported therapies make similar claims. What such claims suggest is that the way to live well, to see what really matters, is through the scientific study of people. But proposals for "better living through science" are still proposals for better living and are not built simply upon scientific data.

Why not? For one thing, an exclusive focus on the empirical tends to occlude the evaluative and the normative, sometimes by stipulating that the evaluative must be derived from the empirical. As we will see in the next chapter, Beck et al. (1979) address concerns that depressed clients may have about shame, self-worth, and fairness in life by critiquing these concepts for their lack of empirical support. As worth and fairness are not empirical concepts, do not name objectively verifiable facts, they should not be given any importance. In the context of treatment, the lack of empirical support for such concepts is the rationale offered to patients for why they should put aside concerns about them. I am skeptical about the merits of this proposal, for most of our evaluative standards (just and unjust, fair and unfair, honorable and ignoble, etc.) have a complex relationship to what can be established empirically that does not allow the direct derivation of one from the other. To demand objective empirical support would undermine many strong evaluations.

An example may help to clarify the issues. Many therapists would agree that there are circumstances in which a patient's complaints of unfairness may be problematic ("it's not fair that my sister is both prettier and smarter than me") and circumstances in which the complaint is justified ("it's not fair that I was told not to take advanced placement math just because I'm a girl"). But the issue here is not that standards of fairness can be established empirically in one case but not in the other. The issue in the first case might be that obsessing about what she cannot change does her harm, fills her with bitterness, has a complex relationship to a broader propensity to envy, or is something she focuses on to avoid another problem. The legitimacy of her complaint about being told not to take AP math isn't founded simply in facts about her previous good grades, but also in a moral principle, in this case, a right to equal educational opportunity regardless of gender. Rights are not discovered through empirical investigation. They are not a part of the natural world that moderns discovered, such as a distant galaxy or a micro-organism. The concept of human rights slowly rose to the point of socio-cultural consensus in a particular historical context as people came to feel that it would be better to live with one another by recognizing these rights.[6] The concept of human rights was part of a proposal for how to live well together that has changed how we live together, not a fact discovered about humans through scientific research. Now that we live within a culture that recognizes universal human rights (at least in principle), it may be clear to us that this is an advance and that to go back would be a loss. We can see that it is better, but this is a very different kind of seeing from discovering a new microbe or astronomical body, for this seeing that it is better is part of what helps to make it real, moves us to act in accord with the notion of human rights, and thus helps to bring into being societies organized around rights. Our discovery that the band of milky light overhead at night is our own galaxy does nothing to change or create that galaxy. We, however, do make and re-make ourselves, individually and collectively, at least in part, through our ideas about who we are and about what matters. We are partly constituted by our self-understanding. In Taylor's (1985a) terms, we are "self-interpreting animals."

Ethical (and political and aesthetic) standards, whether explicitly articulated or enacted in practices, give shape to the way people live their lives. When Beck and colleagues suggest that the treatment of shame, low self-esteem, or bitter clinging to feelings of unfairness can take the form of helping patients to see that there can be no objective foundation for the standards implicit in shame, esteem, and fairness, they are not revealing the "fact" that such standards are illusory. They are proposing a new principle for evaluating standards: don't accept any standards for which there is no clear-cut objective evidence. But no scientific study could show that we should accept this principle. Arguments in favor of it usually take some other form, such as narratives about those who have gotten into trouble trying too hard to meet the demands of an ideal. There are important arguments of this type to be made (and I examine some of them in *Therapeutic Ethics in Context and in Dialogue*). But these are not what we ordinarily think of as empirical arguments. This principle ("no standards without an objective foundation") is itself a strong evaluation that is not based simply on verifiable facts. It is an invitation to live in a way that downgrades to the status of whimsy most of the evaluations that people make (worthy and not, shameful and meritorious, original and derivative, kind and cruel, beautiful and ugly, inspirational and banal). The evaluations that can be supported through objective empirical evidence are few indeed: useful or not for this specific purpose; effective or not at achieving this particular goal. The question about whether a particular purpose or goal is worth pursuing cannot be answered if one adheres to this principle. This principle is a strong evaluation that undermines itself by disallowing strong evaluation.

It seems to be a sort of fact about us that we inevitably live in a space of questions about what matters most. This evaluative space cannot be conflated with questions about how to go about getting what we want. Instead, it entails the assessment of which wants are worth pursuing and which are illusory, self-defeating, alienating, or taking us in a problematic direction. These standards will not be definitively established, with rivals vanquished, the way that science has refuted the geocentric model of the solar system. With regard to notions of human flourishing, science may often have something valuable to contribute, but it won't have the last word.

Strong evaluations are not empirical findings. This has led to the idea of a fact–value dichotomy (for an example in psychology, see Kendler, 2008). According to this view, it is not possible to verify empirically that a value is correct. Therefore, values are not factual, but are seen as part of a separate realm that has nothing to do with what is the case. Evaluations are held to be subjective opinions, culturally or personally shaped preferences about what ought to be that have nothing to do with what is.

There are a number of problems with this distinction being turned into a radical dichotomy (see Putnam, 2002; Taylor, 1985b, pp. 81–90; Taylor, 2003). The validity of the distinction rests upon two claims. The first claim has some merit. Empirical findings, be these everyday perceptual data or the result of scientific research, can provide support for only a narrow range of evaluations. I can see that a watch does not keep accurate time and conclude that it is not a good watch. Toxicology has established that some chemicals are carcinogenic, so exposure to them is bad for human health. But other evaluations have tenuous links to empirical data (at best). "That sonata is sublime." Or: "That congressman's speech was courageous." There are no objective natural facts that can support or disconfirm such evaluations, at least if by "natural facts" one means what one can discern through sensory perception or natural scientific research.

But in order to maintain a strict fact–value dichotomy one needs to add a second claim that has less support. This is the claim that the only facts worthy of the name are those that examine the world, including humans, from a perspective that ignores human significance. People do give reasons for and against aesthetic, moral, political, and spiritual evaluations. Disputes about these matters do not simply come down to "I just like it better." "That sonata demonstrates technical compositional skill, but aesthetically it's rather standard fare, more prosaic than sublime. I can name several other composers who are doing more interesting work." Or: "You call that speech courageous? He's just grandstanding to score points with his own party." Any debate that ensued over these judgments would involve pointing to certain facts (the music of other composers, the history of this politician's career) in the effort to bring one's interlocutor to see things differently. Such facts don't always lead to a straightforward resolution of the argument, like the correction of a faulty sensory perception (in better light I see that the shirt is dark blue, not black). But they are still relevant to the argument. If facts could have no bearing in these debates they would be empty and stir as much passion as an argument about whether strawberry or chocolate ice cream were better. The latter dispute is about matters of taste that can't be rationally justified.

Further, it is questionable whether we can study the human world without bringing some evaluative assumptions into the work. This is clear in therapeutic theorizing. When Beck argues that one can overcome various psychological problems by adopting rational thinking, or Freud argues for an improvement in the quality of life and a decrease in neurosis through altering the repression of sexual and aggressive impulses, each is joining together ethical aims (about rationality or the value of honestly facing who one is) to ideas about psychological functioning. The issue isn't that there is a radical disjunction of facts and values, but that in the realm of strong evaluation, of considerations about what is truly important in life, facts and values intermingle and influence each other and are examined and understood in the light of each other. As an example, consider how Shedler (2010) responds to the claim that psychodynamic therapy is less effective than other types of therapy. He not only presents data from research that shows that it is as effective, but questions whether the standard measure of better therapy should be symptom reduction. How did we come to decide that symptom reduction is more important than the development of other kinds of psychological resources to live more fully and richly?

Questions inevitably arise as to which facts really matter, and matter for the sake of what end. Facts about people can take on different significances when viewed through the lens of different pictures of human flourishing. What does it mean to defend or argue for a proposal about human flourishing? Can such arguments have validity? Can there be "perceptions" regarding what is the case about where the good lies? To see ethically, to see that compassion is the appropriate response to suffering, or that self-restraint can be an important component of good character, is not like seeing empirically. Ethical perceptions (including the two just referenced) can be argued for and critiqued, but they are not what we think of as empirical or scientific. They do not appear in a world viewed through a scientific lens that abstracts from human meanings. They occur only within a world that is already ethically oriented. Much of what we mean by empirical seeing (certainly the scientific sort) does not take place in an ethical world. It is an examination of how things are apart from the valences that strong evaluations give to the world. This is true even if that scientific examination is initiated in order to improve well-being. For example, research that establishes the effectiveness of a chemotherapy will not answer ethical questions about how to balance the value of extending one's life against the decline in quality of life that comes with the treatment. Ethical questions like this require a different framework of assessment.

Within an ethical world it does make sense to speak of someone having a keen "eye" for what is right or valuable, even if this is a skilled seeing that needs to be developed, and that can vary across persons and contexts. It is akin to an aesthetic perception, like hearing that one performance of a jazz standard was lackluster while another had depth and originality. Indeed, this sort of aesthetic seeing is closely related to ethical seeing in the sense I am using the term here, for devotion to an aesthetic ideal can be a strong evaluation. This example also indicates the difficulties inherent in such perceptions—they are dependent on familiarity and experience with the material, are culturally located, and can be made on the basis of standards that change over time. But that does not mean that there are no facts of the matter here. In the world of human significance, seeing the facts of the matter requires the development of an individual's skills of attunement, skills that can, individually and collectively, undergo further development, challenge, or decay.

I take up a more detailed examination of the possibilities for ethical truth in *Therapeutic Ethics in Context and in Dialogue*. In the next few chapters I describe in more detail the sense in which the psychotherapies promote ethical ideals.

Notes

1 All the names here are pseudonyms, and the therapy descriptions are composites.
2 In *Therapeutic Ethics in Context and in Dialogue* I examine the origins of various therapeutic aims and ideals in the history of the modern West, following the work of Charles Taylor (1989, 2007b).

3 Taylor (1995b, 2007a) contrasts his claim regarding the interconnection of fundamental moral obligations and ideas about a good life with the position of philosophers who keep the two distinct, such as Habermas and Rawls.
4 For examples, see de Waal (2006) and Rowlands (2012).
5 In Rowlands's (2012) terms, some animals are capable of being moral subjects,
   but not moral agents.
6 See Taylor's (1986) short overview of the development of the concept of rights in
   the West.

3   Therapeutic Ethics in "Technical" Therapies

Introduction: The Interweaving of the Psychological and the Ethical

The claim that all therapies embody an ethic needs to meet a fundamental challenge: psychotherapists certainly have ideas about what would be better for their patients, but these ideas have little to do with ethics. It is not good to have a broken arm. Or if it is broken, it is good for it to heal properly. Does that make an orthopedist an ethicist, a proponent of a specific picture of a good life? Similarly, therapists are not proposing an ethic when they agree with their patients that it is good not to be depressed, addicted to drugs, tormented by accusatory voices, or constantly in fear of the next panic attack. If this is an ethic, it is simply an ethic of health that is shared by all. Whether someone is a conscientious seeker after the good of others, a simple hedonist, a Marxist revolutionary, or a fundamentalist Christian, they no more want to be depressed than they want a broken arm. The values of psychological health are neutral with regard to what we call ethics.

The quickest response to such a challenge is to point out that the project to portray human problems in terms of behaviors, symptoms, and disorders as one would in orthopedic medicine is itself an ethical proposal. It is a recommendation to treat the difficulties people bring to therapy as having a distinct causal history, delimited meaning, and treatment indications that render them amenable to the approach of applying interventions to disorders. This is an ethical proposal in the sense that it is offered as an alternative to other ethical proposals. The fundamentalist Christian may view hostile voices as evidence of demonic possession. The conscientious political activist who is dedicated to social justice may believe that bouts of depression are an acceptable price to pay for frequently frustrated efforts to alleviate suffering and oppression in a world resistant to change. The hedonist may be willing to accept the risks of addiction, even of overdose and death, for the sake of the pleasure the drug brings. When therapists propose an alternative framework for these experiences as symptoms of treatable disorders they are changing the context of meaning for them. Accepting this alternative framework will change the shape of patients' experiences and influence patients to revamp their picture of themselves. To challenge patients' ideas about evil, self-sacrifice, and pleasure is to engage in ethical work. The fact that the alternative is offered as a more realistic, scientific, or pragmatic approach for how to live a good life does not make it non-ethical. Nor does therapeutic work become less ethical if the patient comes to therapy already accepting the framework offered by the therapist. In that case, the therapist is not converting the patient to a new vision but building on a shared picture of how to improve life that sustains and enacts their common understanding of human flourishing.

While I am arguing for a distinction between the aims of medicine and the aims of therapy, I recognize that some could make physical health a central component of their ethics, seeing it as essential to a good life. But to do so is to do something very different from seeking treatment for a broken arm. Consider people who are careful about how they eat, who avoid dangerous activities that involve risk of injury, and who are careful to get the exercise they feel is necessary to stay healthy. Someone who followed this course might have the sense that what matters most is living a long life so that one can continue to experience everyday joys and pleasures. By contrast, there are those who value health for the sake of living at a peak of physical accomplishment or endurance. For an ultra-marathon runner, health may be a prerequisite to or component of testing one's limits, with the risk of injury even being integral to an ideal of courageous pursuit of physical challenge as a means to prove one's mettle, to push past fears and exhaustion, or to feel a high that comes with athletic exertion. Both of these motivations for health may result in being healthy according to standard medical assessment. But these two people are living different lives based on different visions of what constitutes a good life.

Some might use these two examples to reinforce the distinction between ethics and therapy. A doctor may well judge both these people to be healthy, but that does not authorize an opinion on which version of healthy living is better than the other. The doctor's expertise does not extend beyond providing guidance regarding a healthy lifestyle. The doctor has no right to instruct patients on other details of their lives. Likewise, a therapist's job is to help patients attain a basic level of psychological health. What patients then do with this improved state is not the therapist's concern. To bring a patient out of a deep depression or to help a patient to maintain his recovery from addiction does not license a therapist to instruct patients about what to do with their better mood or sobriety. Therapists treat depression and addiction. It's not their job to change other aspects of patients' lives that may be deeply meaningful to them, such as their careers, marital status, religion, or political affiliation.

However, it is one thing to be respectful of people's beliefs and practices. It is another to claim that therapists will have no influence on someone's fundamental views because the psychological is walled off from the ethical. The psychological realm is not completely contained within its own domain but is influenced by and has links to broader aspects of patients' lives. Patients often come to therapy with problems that are intricately linked to their understanding of what is most important in life. Consider the patient with an eating disorder whose life is centered on the ideal of being thin or the narcissist who protects his sense of worth by demeaning others. It is likely that changes in these psychological problems will involve changes to what these patients have hitherto considered of utmost importance in their lives.

Or consider an example that is not clearly linked to a diagnosable mental disorder. A freshman at a prestigious university is overwhelmed by how much more difficult the work is now than it was in high school. He feels shaken in his self-esteem as a core component of his identity is put in question.

> I was always the smartest kid in my class in grade school and high school. Now I'm about average. I don't know how to be average, and I miss being the one whom others looked up to, sometimes even envied. I guess I must admit I liked being envied. That I'm not very special is hard for me to take. Being the smartest meant a lot to me. I'm not the funniest, my family doesn't have a lot of money, and I don't think I'm good-looking. Nothing sets me apart anymore. I feel like a nobody.

His therapy may well entail re-thinking his assumption that in order to be worthwhile he must have some status ("the smart one") that sets him above others. He may find himself reconsidering whether it is so important to be extraordinary, whether that is necessary for a decent life.

Or consider an obsessional woman who begins to see in therapy that the fixed routines in her life isolate her from others and function to protect and distract her from various doubts and anxieties. Some of these routines are evident in her religious practice, and some of the doubts are about her religion. As she begins to ease up on the obsessional demands she places upon herself, she may be less rigid in her daily routines, religious and otherwise. She may also allow herself to contemplate more fully the religious doubts that she has previously been afraid to entertain. Perhaps this will lead to wholesale questioning of her faith. It may also lead to a deeper, less brittle faith as she comes to see doubt as integral to faith. In either case, the psychological change in her obsessional style can have an impact on her fundamental beliefs and practices.[1]

So the distinction one can readily make between physical health and one's conception of what makes life worthwhile is not easily transposed to the psychological arena. There is something about psychological problems, in themselves, that links with broader life meanings in ways that biological problems do not. What do I mean by "in themselves"? Examination of a broken arm won't reveal broader life meanings except in the manner of a sign. In the course of an examination, a doctor may say to a patient: "This appears to be the result of a blow. Were you in an accident? Were you hit with something?" Perhaps the doctor is wondering about an abusive spouse. Here the injury may point to some broader life meaning, ultimately even to a desperate project to rescue others that keeps the patient in an abusive relationship. But the injury is only an indicator of a possible link to what matters most to this patient. Examination of an X-ray film will not confirm it. For that the doctor will need to talk to the patient.

One might object that a change of example would paint a different picture. A doctor sees what appear to be self-inflicted cuts on a patient's arm, as well as the scars from older cuts on her thighs and abdomen. The possibility of borderline pathology immediately comes to mind. Nevertheless, we're still at the level of a sign, of a possible diagnostic marker. Consider how the patient's understanding or perspective on the cutting changes the nature of the problem. When asked to explain how she got these cuts, one patient may answer: "Oh, I had a fight with my mother last night and I couldn't get her to shut up." She then shrugs as if to suggest that it's no big deal. She also is apparently unaware that what she has just said doesn't explain much to the person asking about the cuts. Contrast this with a patient who says that she cut herself because the voices tell her to do so when the devil puts evil thoughts into her head. The cuts themselves won't reveal differences in psychopathology. The patient's understanding (or misunderstanding) of the problem does, for such understandings are partly constitutive of the nature of the problem. There is no equivalent to this in the medical evaluation of a broken arm. Whether the patient believes a broken arm is due to a fall off a bicycle or an evil spell won't differentiate a compound from a hairline fracture. Nor will those different medical diagnoses reveal anything about the patient's practices of bike riding or voodoo.

Psychological problems are partly constituted by patients' perspectives on those problems in a way that medical problems are not. Psychological phenomena become what they are through how they are understood. Self-understandings are part of a connected network of meanings, some of which will be more explicitly ethical. Psychopathology can be intricately interwoven with, and partly constituted by, patients' beliefs about their problems, with how they see themselves in relationship to others, and with expectations, aims, and ideals that guide their lives. For example, a patient struggling with alcoholism is wracked with guilt and regret over having alienated his family. In his mind, his drinking is both an effort to numb the guilt and a punishment he deserves (he knows his drinking is destroying him). Further inquiry reveals that he grew up in a family in which he was told from an early age that he resembled his father "and would probably wind up a no-good drunk just like him." This was the assessment of his mother, who was embittered over being abandoned by her husband. Is the patient's alcoholism a gift ("Is this what you want me to be, Mom?") that is also an act of revenge ("See what you've done to me, Mom")? Is this a story the patient tells to justify himself, to assuage his guilt, to push responsibility onto her? Maybe it is all of the above, and more.

To intervene therapeutically with this person will bring about a shift (in some manner, to some degree) in how he understands himself, or lives his life and engages with others in the light of certain aims. This will entail a shift in his sense of what matters. This man may continue to feel guilty about the havoc he has wrought in the lives of those he loves, but after treatment he may take his guilt as part of a larger platform that helps him to move in a new direction, perhaps through a process of making amends in a twelve-step program. Such a change is a change in this person's orientation toward and understanding of what is possible in life, what is worthwhile, and where he places himself in relation to this new perspective. Such a change in perspective is a change in ethics.

The fact that alcoholism and its treatment implicate a perspective on what makes life worthwhile makes the disease model of alcoholism less than fully satisfactory (however helpful it may be to combat social stigma, and however much evidence is accumulated regarding underlying neurobiology and genetics). It also means that a picture of alcoholism (or depression, panic disorder, etc.) that models it on medical disorders misses something important. A healed broken arm may make it possible to return to a valued form of life (for example, as a professional athlete). But a healed arm is not a way of living. By contrast, for alcoholics to be in recovery is to live a different form of life. Depressed patients who have been excessively self-critical improve their mood by changing the way they evaluate themselves, and in so doing change the way they live their lives. They change the sense of what to expect of themselves and now see prior perfectionist demands as destructive.

I am not suggesting that medical and psychological/ethical issues exist in self-enclosed realms. One can certainly *affect* the other. Chronic physical problems can cause depression, for example. People with mental disorders tend to have poorer physical health (see Niles & O'Donovan, 2019). Further, medical problems can be a spur to changing how one lives. A heart attack may prompt someone to engage in heart-healthy behaviors. This change may be done simply for the sake of living, in order not to die from another heart attack. But this only expresses the sense that life is worth living, not what makes life worthwhile. In another case, a heart attack may prompt someone to re-evaluate their ethics, their sense of what is really important in life. It is not unusual for someone to ask questions after a serious medical illness about the relative importance of work, family, community involvement, or an avocation. But such a re-evaluation is triggered by the emotional impact of the illness as a forceful reminder of mortality. It is not a treatment for it the way that a patient's embrace of life changes in recovery is a treatment for alcoholism. The treatment of psychological disorders can easily involve intervening in beliefs (some more implicit than fully articulated), wishes, and disappointments regarding living life well, not just living. Psychological problems are not simply impediments to someone's efforts to pursue their goals. They often implicate or embody notions about what goals are worth pursuing and what makes them so. Interventions that treat such disorders can change a patient's evaluations about which goals are worthy of pursuit, and why.

Psychological problems can become de-contextualized, disentangled from ethics in some cases. Horwitz and Wakefield (2007) argue that disconnection from context is what distinguishes the mental disorder of depression from the ordinary (if sometimes intense and even debilitating) sadness that occurs in response to stressors. Ordinary sadness has an expectable connection to "losses of intimate attachments, low or declining social status, or the failure to achieve desired goals" (p. 219) and tends to be self-remitting over time. By contrast, depressive disorder occurs either without an initiating stressor, or is out of proportion to the stressor, or becomes detached from the stressor (lasts long after the stressor is past). The person with a depressive disorder has been captured by a mood and accompanying symptoms that are disconnected from the circumstances of the person's life. On this picture of depression, successful treatment entails bringing the person back to ethics, back into a life shaped by practices and aims that constitute a framework for the effort to live well.

If this distinction between the mental disorder of depression and ordinary sadness is valid, does it map onto a requirement for different types of treatment? Perhaps ordinary sadness in response to a loss or stressor benefits from a therapy that helps the patient to re-connect to a meaningful good, a therapy that promotes an ethical vision of living well. And perhaps the mental disorder of depression requires intervention into more fundamental factors that operate at a level "beneath" ethics (for example, at a biological level, or at the level of basic cognitive or learning processes). The fact is, we don't know if these two forms of dysphoria require different treatments because, as Horwitz and Wakefield point out, current research has not paid any attention to the distinction. Studies of treatment have lumped the two together. But even if we had research to support differential treatment, it is not clear that this would point to the value of a therapy for depressive disorder that operates outside the ethical realm. The psychotherapies seem to inevitably incorporate ethics in a way that would make it difficult to identify a therapy as "psychological but not ethical." The following examples are intended to illustrate this.

Ethics in Technical Therapies

Exposure Therapy for Eating Disorders

If psychological phenomena often have a connection to ethical aims, then therapeutic intervention in psychological problems can have an impact on patients' ethical views. Further, therapies that are designed to treat mental disorders often include ethical perspectives as well. I would like to illustrate this link between therapy and ethics by showing how it is present even in therapies that aim to address circumscribed problems by technical means. In these days of manualized treatments it is not difficult to find examples of such therapies. Glasofer et al. (2016) present a clear description of a treatment for anorexia nervosa that attempts to decrease the fear of eating through exposure and response prevention (EXRP). EXRP has been successfully used to treat obsessive–compulsive disorder (see Barlow, 2002; Franklin & Foa, 2014). Exposure in this context means directing patients to be in direct contact with situations or objects that have typically provoked both anxious avoidance and compulsive efforts to ritualistically counter a risk associated with being in the presence of the object. For example, someone who has obsessional fears of microbial contamination may be asked to hold the doorknob in a public building for a sustained period of time and then is not allowed to engage in compulsive handwashing afterward. (Needless to say, such techniques need to be modified during a health crisis in which there are realistic concerns about contamination.) Extended periods of exposure to the anxiety-provoking stimulus without the utilization of countering rituals allow the patient to learn that the anxiety will dissipate even without their compulsive efforts to undo the imagined contamination. Through the repeated experience of such exposures patients learn that compulsions are not necessary to reduce anxiety or to prevent the feared outcome. The adaptation of Glasofer et al. (2016) for anorexia nervosa is intended to do something similar for the fear of eating. The experience of decreased anxiety through repeated exposure, combined with recognition that the feared consequences of eating do not occur, diminishes both the anxious phobic response and the need for compulsive control over eating.

Glasofer et al. (2016) present a detailed description of a case study. Central to the patient's fears in this case was the belief that if her eating was not restricted she would experience unending weight gain. A series of exposure exercises were developed in collaboration with the patient. There were several rituals and avoidant behaviors regarding food and eating that became the basis for an exposure hierarchy. The authors detail the particular ways the patient behaved toward food and how the therapist carefully explored the nuances of the patient's anxieties, her catastrophic fantasies, her hyper-focus on feeling full, and her avoidant behaviors.

The therapist carefully attended to the relationship with her patient while frequently pushing the patient to engage in difficult activities. She repeatedly worked to elicit the patient's endorsement of therapeutic procedures. She patiently explained the rationale for the treatment and offered support to continue the difficult work that the therapy required. The therapist writes in her article of being "in there" with the patient, carefully attending to and encouraging the patient not to avoid her most intense fears. This required a focus on the particulars of the patient's fears. The therapy was not a generic hierarchy of exposures that could be applied to any patient, nor would any patient's fears about food have taken exactly the same form. These elements of attention to the state of the alliance, support for the patient's effort when treatment becomes difficult, encouragement to face what is emotionally distressing, providing a rationale for treatment, and attending to the particulars of the patient's problems—all these are common to many therapies.

But beyond these common factors lies the specific technique of exposure. The role of support is not to simply reassure but to encourage the patient to deliberately do that which will increase her anxiety, that which her fearful inclinations would lead her to avoid. One might describe this treatment as a program of planned acts of courage. The aim is to decrease fear and increase the patient's sense of self-control. Instead of the effort to control or diminish the urge to eat, the patient is learning to control or diminish her fear of eating. The message of the treatment might be: "You can master your fear of food. You don't have to let your fear rule you. Let me show you how." At the beginning of treatment this message may not even be heard the way it is presented by the therapist. The patient may see what is coming as: "I am going to have my control over my eating taken away from me." The presentation of the rationale for treatment, the therapist's efforts at collaborative engagement, the encouragement to proceed when anxious—all this might be seen as the effort to bring this fearful person far enough along into the exposure exercises for her to experience the benefits herself. The hoped for outcome is not simply decreased symptoms at the end of this short treatment, but an increased sense of efficacy and autonomy, a capacity to master that which had previously mastered her.

It should be clear that even this treatment that utilizes specific procedures to decrease a circumscribed set of symptoms includes more than effective interventions. The therapist provides supportively tough encouragement to be courageous in the face of fear, attention to the collaborative state of the relationship, and efforts to enhance the patient's understanding of and control over a specific problem. The specific technical interventions support the broader goals of enhancing the patient's autonomy and self-efficacy. Even this technical therapy focused on specific symptoms promotes a particular vision of living well by introducing the patient to that vision through therapeutic practices that enact it. As Miller (2004) puts it, "Whatever the therapeutic goal, therapy consists of exposing the client to small, regular doses of that end" (p. 91). The ends of this therapy cannot be characterized simply as the application of scientifically based techniques to reduce or remove symptoms. The double-blind provision of a pharmacotherapy for her symptoms might come closer to meriting such a description. But here an appeal is made to the patient, a justification (treatment rationale) is offered, a sense of shared bond is built upon the experience of working together, and an effort is made to foster a wish in the patient to feel more in charge of her life. Understanding, collaboration, courage, autonomy: all these may have some relationship to therapeutic efficacy, to achieving a circumscribed goal (decreased symptoms of anorexia nervosa). But if someone proposed to treat the disorder without enhancing these (or some other) fundamental values, virtues, or ethical aims, would it still be recognizable as psychotherapy? Imagine a future biological intervention more sophisticated than today's pharmacotherapy, an intervention that changes symptomatology by direct neuro-chemical modulation. Perhaps (if such an idea doesn't remain in the realm of science fiction, as I am inclined to believe) this would be entirely effective without any appeal to or engagement of the patient in the ethical realm. It clearly would not be psychotherapy.

Ethical notions of what makes life better are part and parcel of even symptom-focused treatments. Alongside the question of the relative efficacy of different techniques lie questions about broader ethical aims. In this case, exposure operates as part of a call to courage in the service of self-efficacy and autonomy. Too often the ethical aims of therapy are overlooked or seen as mere means to the more "substantial" aim of treating pathology. The treatment of pathology is essential to what therapy is about—but it is interwoven with and partly composed of ethical aims that are not separable from what are proposed as the proven efficacious elements of the treatment.

Cognitive Therapy for Depression

Different treatments (or a given treatment at different points in the course of therapy) may emphasize different ethical ideas, different pictures of well-being. *Cognitive Therapy of Depression* (Beck et al., 1979) is a classic work in the movement to systematize and manualize the psychotherapies. As such, it has contributed not only to the dissemination and popularization of cognitive-behavioral therapy, but also to research efforts to establish its efficacy.

The role that this book has played in the project to establish efficacious treatment for depression should not obscure the fact that it also promotes a number of ethical ideas. This therapy is not simply offered as an effective means to treat depression. It also promotes efficacy as a value to live by, as a key ingredient of human well-being. In this regard, it is significant that this treatment is "offered" to the patient, not "delivered." The authors stress that this therapy cannot be applied mechanistically but should be understood in humanistic terms (Beck et al., 1979, p. 36). This therapy does not aim to convince patients of something on the basis of the therapist's authority. Patients are encouraged to assess, challenge, and test the tenets and practices of the therapy to see if they make sense and work for them. In fact, one could say that this therapy partly consists of helping patients to develop the skills to assess and test ideas: their own, but also those the therapist offers. At the ethical core of this therapy is a belief in the value of searching for evidence for what one believes and abandoning views contradicted by the evidence. Patients are encouraged to take a scientific attitude toward understanding their problems. Science does not stand passive before aspects of life that may seem mysterious and overwhelming. Rather, science tries to grasp how things work in order to convert "mysteries into problems, because problems, unlike mysteries, are designed to be solved" (p. 273).

However, cognitive therapy is not focused on teaching patients the value of a hypothesis-testing stance as an abstract principle. Its practical aim is to assist patients in applying such principles to the specifics of their symptoms, their problematic cognitions, and their fundamental assumptions. The goal is to help patients develop a sense of where particular errors lie in their thinking. As an exercise in skill building rather than in imparting information, the therapist is not to lecture the patient, but to ask questions and offer alternative perspectives for the patient's consideration. For example, in the transcript of a session with a suicidal patient the authors make clear that everything is up for consideration, including the advantages and disadvantages of killing herself (Beck et al., 1979, p. 230). Such questions are examined not in general terms, but by looking at the particular reasons the patient believes her life is hopeless. The patient is asked to look for evidence supporting or contradicting her sense that she can't be happy without a romantic relationship, that she has in fact found nothing of satisfaction in her life lately, or that she has not had any variations in mood but felt unremitting despair (pp. 229–243).

The belief in the value of evidence includes a belief that people can find relevant and helpful evidence, that the world in general and their psychological problems in particular can be understood, and that thinking things through will provide access to an "objective reality" (Beck et al., 1979, p. 235) in which they can act more effectively to attain what they want. Indeed, it is what people want that takes precedence over what others think or what they have been told they should want. Prescriptions for how people should live their lives may be part of the problem, in part because these prescriptions are often imposed by others. Further, it is difficult to find evidence to support normative "shoulds." Issues of fairness (p. 258), self-worth (p. 266), feelings of shame (p. 282), and questions about hidden motivations that contribute to depression (p. 304) all operate outside the realm of that which is empirically supportable. Such issues and feelings represent a kind of quicksand in which it is difficult to find one's footing. People need the solid ground of evidence in order to move toward what they want.

Patients know what they want, to no longer be depressed, and the therapist's job is to help them get there (Beck et al., 1979, p. 280). Hence, therapists have an ethic for their work, too, a recommended stance toward the patient. This stance communicates a particular message: "Yes, this is difficult, but I have some ways to help you. I am ready to work with you to change things and want to invite you to work with me to make things better. Indeed, it is only through our both working on this together that any headway will be made. You can be assured that I am not going to sit back and let you flounder until you find your way, or until some mysterious change occurs that neither you nor I can actively bring about. We are going to chart a path together, complete with exercises and experiments to be done here and at home, always ready to change course as the results of our work together dictate."

The scientific ethos of cognitive therapy is linked to another fundamental value: autonomy. Part of patients' problems may be linked to a tendency to let others do their thinking for them (Beck et al., 1979, p. 246). The project to critically assess beliefs not only is more likely to bring one's beliefs into line with reality, but also allows patients to develop a degree of independence from others, no longer taking someone else's word as final without testing it themselves.

There is evidence that cognitive therapy can treat depression. But as the authors of this text make clear, it is not through a mechanistic application of techniques, but through the respectful and persistent engagement of the patient in a series of activities and exercises that embody and strengthen the patient's capacity for empirical thinking, for challenging previously unquestioned assumptions, combined with an affirmation of the patient's own desires and the development of a critical distance from their own and others' expectations. This therapy embodies a particular stance toward oneself and others that proposes a particular picture of a flourishing life. It promotes an ethic of scientific detachment and autonomous individualism based in the pursuit of one's own desires, combined with a robust skepticism toward that which cannot be empirically established. It is not simply a technical means to a circumscribed end.

Conclusion

Even therapies that are promoted as scientific interventions to change well-defined pathology include implicit ethics or conceptions of human flourishing. Therapies may draw allegiance from practitioners, researchers, and patients not simply because they have been shown to work, but because they embody an appealing ethic. Some scientifically minded therapists may be uncomfortable with justifying a therapy on the grounds that it promotes a particular set of ideas about how to live well. On the contrary, I think it is an unavoidable aspect of being human that no amount of scientific analysis could or should expunge. We never live completely outside of questions regarding what makes life worthwhile (including the question of whether it is).

If ethical views are present even in technical therapies that claim to be grounded in psychological science, then the presence of ethics is even more obvious when one examines the full range of therapeutic orientations. One does not have to read between the lines of much therapeutic writing to find frequent appeals to a picture of human well-being. Rogers's (1951) client-centered therapy clearly aims to enhance the capacity to be true to one's "organismic values" and to resist succumbing to the social demands to modify such values. For Rogers there is a true self that the patient can be assisted to discover beneath the distortions created by familial and social pressures. This self does not need to be changed but only set free, which is part of the rationale for the non-directive quality of the therapy. Patients need to be given space within which to find themselves, not to be made better according to an external standard, whether that of society or of the therapist.

With existential therapy the ethical realm is present in the very name and defining concerns of the therapy. Yalom's (1980) therapy promotes the ultimate value of a more direct confrontation with existential givens of life: the knowledge that we will die, the dilemmas and demands of freedom, the pain of isolation and meaninglessness. Facing issues such as these does not suggest that flourishing consists of comfortable contentment. What is on offer is a picture of a fuller life that is lived honestly and courageously through coming to grips with difficult existential facts that Yalom argues are inevitable features of the human condition.

Examples could be taken from many other varieties of therapy. There would be both overlap and distinctiveness among the pictures of well-being, of how we are called by them to shape or orient our lives for the better. My concern here is not to survey all such views but to illustrate that much of what is in dispute between the therapies can be understood as rival pictures of therapeutic benefit that are rooted in different ideas about what we should aspire to in living our lives, not just in changing our symptoms. Such differences even appear in closely related therapies. In Chapter 4 I turn to psychoanalysis to examine how the differences between its competing sub-schools may be understood in terms of their distinct ethical orientations.

Note

1 For a more detailed example of therapeutic influence on religious belief and practice, see Slife et al. (2016).

4 Different Therapies, Different Ethics

The Example of Psychoanalysis

It is difficult to conceive of a therapy that does not include some ideas about human flourishing. This is true even of therapies that claim to be straightforward applications of scientific principles to alleviate narrowly defined problems. Further, one can distinguish therapies from one another on the basis of their distinct conceptions of flourishing. Different views of human well-being clarify part of what is at stake between different therapies. That is, the various therapies are not simply different means to bring about an agreed upon end of psychological health. They promote different pictures of what it is to be psychologically healthy. Indeed, they even disagree about whether the term "psychological health" is the appropriate heading under which to subsume their various aims.

The role that differences in ethics play in differentiating the therapies is evident even if one looks at closely related therapies, for example, different schools of psychoanalysis. Proponents of these schools often argue about whether their picture of psychodynamics, mind, or subjectivity is correct, whether it accurately captures the subject matter of psychoanalytic theory and practice. Advocates of the respective schools sometimes claim to have more evidence in support of their perspective, pointing to research from infant observation, process research, clinical case studies, the social sciences, the humanities, arts, and literature. However, careful examination of different analytic schools reveals another way to conceptualize their disagreements. They are not simply arguing about whose theory has better evidence to support its picture of human subjectivity but are expressing allegiance to ideas about how to live well that are implicit in their respective schools' theories and practices. I want to illustrate this by examining three versions of psychoanalysis: Paul Gray's ego psychology, Bruce Fink's Lacanian psychoanalysis, and Stephen Mitchell's relational analysis. An exposition of psychoanalytic aims will also broaden the picture of therapeutic ethics presented in Chapter 3 by examining an orientation that is often contrasted with cognitive-behavioral treatment.

Paul Gray's Ego-Psychology

One of the more striking aspects of Paul Gray's writing on psychoanalysis is the clarity of his exposition. On finishing his book *The Ego and Analysis of Defense* (1994) there is little difficulty picturing how he worked, the ways of doing analysis that he avoided (when possible), and the rationale for both. This quality of his writing matches his recommendations for analytic practice. A central aim of what he calls "essential psychoanalysis" (as opposed to psychodynamic psychotherapy) is to deepen patients' understanding of how their minds work. This is done not by telling patients, not by interpreting *for* them, but by showing patients that which they can see themselves regarding their efforts to deflect from anxiety-provoking material in session. Gray wants to help patients develop a clarity of understanding about their defensive functions. He aims not so much to change patients through interventions (whether they come in the form of interpretations or through the therapeutic relationship) as to bring patients to an understanding of the ways they have been involuntarily avoiding giving expression to various libidinal or aggressive impulses. Coming to see this, and to see that the reasons for restricting the expression of drive derivatives no longer hold, the patient will then be in a position to choose what to do with those impulses. The choice will be freer because it will be made on the basis of a clearer understanding that the risks of drive expression are not what they were (or were imagined to be) when the defenses were first instituted in childhood.

Gray summarizes the analyst's task succinctly (1994, pp. 91–92). The analyst listens for aggressive or libidinal feelings or actions reported in the patient's speech or present in the patient's manner of speaking (for example, in an affectively charged expression of anger or desire). The analyst points to instances in which the patient reacts to the appearance of these drive derivatives by inhibiting, steering away from, or contradicting their direct expression.

As an example of calling the patient's attention to defensive action consider the following:

> You were speaking angrily about your husband's coldness to you and then abruptly shifted to talking of his conscientious attention to the children, of what a dutiful father he is. As you did so, all the anger dropped out of your voice. There was something about expressing your anger so forcefully here that felt dangerous and you quickly tried to take it back or soften it.

Gray presents more complex examples in which the drive derivative is directed at both the analyst and figures in the patient's life and is defended against on multiple levels. He writes (1994, pp. 13–16) of a patient who displaced his anger toward the analyst by talking about a recent argument with his wife and then focused his description of the argument upon his efforts to control his anger. The analyst notes how the patient would not let himself re-experience his anger at his wife in the session. Instead he tells the story in such a way as to focus on efforts to control his anger *then*, in order not to feel the anger *now*—something feels dangerous about bringing his anger into the room.

The aim of such analytic work is to help patients begin to see their defenses in action. Further inquiry may explore the nature of the danger that the patient associates with the open expression of libidinal or aggressive feelings. Gray is alert to patients transferentially displacing the censure of their own superegos onto the analyst. Patients fantasize that the analyst will disapprove of their impulses just as childhood authorities did. Analysts can help to drain the power of such transference fantasies by assisting patients to notice the way they shift away from certain topics or ways of expressing them, then exploring the felt sense of risk that led to the defensive action. Gray directs patients' attention to aspects of their thoughts, feelings, and speech that they can see unfolding in their immediate experience in the session. He does not offer insights into unconscious influences that are beyond their grasp. The aim is to reduce the need to engage in involuntary inhibition and defense by analyzing the irrational nature of the implicit assumption that freer emotional expression is dangerous.

Gray's critiques of other ways of doing analysis further highlight the distinctiveness of his approach.

Against Depth Interpretation

The type of depth interpretation that Gray is critical of is one that bypasses the patient's awareness. Analysts may be correct when they suggest that unconscious libidinal or aggressive wishes explain patients' actions, speech, dreams, or symptoms. But if patients are not in a position to see these wishes, analysts are short-circuiting what would be most beneficial to their patients— a strengthened capacity to see for themselves how they defend against drive derivatives. Further, if patients assent to an interpretation without seeing it themselves (perhaps it just seems plausible) they may be assenting in order to please the analyst, to avoid conflict, or because they are invested in seeing the analyst as having a wisdom or expertise they do not have. That is, this assent will simply enact that which deserves analysis. Attention to a patient's response to an interpretation is recommended by analysts of various schools for a variety of reasons. Gray's particular concern is that analysis will be less successful if interpretations point to that which is outside of patients' awareness than if they point to defensive activities that patients can observe themselves. Once patients come to see their defensive maneuvers, and recognize their roots in childhood situations that are no longer pertinent, whatever has been defended against will be available for patients to express if and how they choose. To be able to see and dismantle defensive activity is all that is necessary. What has been defended against will then show itself, enabling patients to make more mature and rational decisions about what to do with it.

Against the Therapeutic Use of the Transference

Gray is critical of analysts who would use the transference rather than analyze it. He is wary of the idea that an analyst can use a patient's transference in order to sway the patient to acknowledge the truth of an interpretation. He sees in this idea a return to the pre-analytic use of suggestion in treatment, a move that is to be avoided because it undermines the patient's autonomy. This idea of using transference is an old one in psychoanalysis, and he cites (1994, p. 38) as an example Freud's (1917/1963, pp. 445 & 455) reference in the *Introductory Lectures* to enlisting the aid of positive transference in order to disarm the ego's resistance to interpretation. Gray sees an authoritarian element here, an effort to influence patients emotionally rather than to show them something rationally.

Gray sees a similar problem with what he calls "therapeutic action by internalization" (1994, p. 52). He rejects Strachey's idea that analysis works through "the gradual replacement of the primitive superego by the incorporation of the contemporary image of the analyst" (p. 52—he is referencing Strachey, 1934). Gray reads Strachey as characterizing the analytic process as a series of small increments of introjection of the analyst. He cites with approval Fenichel's (1937/1954, p. 24) critique: "I think he [Strachey] uses the concept of 'introjection' in a wider sense than is legitimate. When I recognize that what someone says is right, it does not necessarily mean that I have introjected him." Here again is the contrast between an emotional process of identification with or introjection of the analyst and a reasoned coming to see *with* the analyst that something is the case. For Gray, the most important thing that patients can come to see is that they are engaging in some form of defense.

Nor is Gray happy with the notion of the analyst as offering a more benign, affectionate, or approving presence to counteract the patient's punitive superego. Gray recommends that the analyst adopt a non-critical professional stance, not an affectionate parental attitude. When patients operate under the image of their analyst as someone who permissively likes and approves of them, they may be less likely to censor at least some of their thoughts. But this will be situation specific, and does not help patients develop the skills to discern and undo the defensive activities they are likely to continue in environments that seem less permissive, including moments in analysis in which the fantasy of the analyst as warmly approving feels threatened. Further, sensing that they have won the analyst's affection or approval may have the opposite effect, leading to an increased carefulness about what they say so as not to lose that approval.

Against a Focus on the Patient's Life

Patients talk about the details of their lives, current and past, about what happened and what they fantasized, remembered, or dreamt. For Gray, the analyst's focus should not be on the content of such talk, on what happened, was done, fantasized or dreamt, but on the telling of it (or steering away from the telling of it) in the session. When analysts focus on the content, on how patients avoid the expression of aggressive or erotic feelings toward persons in their lives, patients may come to believe that what their analyst wants is for them to live their lives differently, to change their relationships with others, or to be a different sort of person. Under such influence patients can come to feel pressured to bring their behaviors outside the session into conformity with what the analyst seems to want. This departure from analytic neutrality undermines patient autonomy.

Gray recommends instead that analysts' interventions be directed to how patients change the way they talk or the content of what they say because of anxiety about revealing something to the analyst. Patients are directed to understand the occurrence and nature of their anxiety, and how it derailed their speech. Patients are being directed to pay attention to how their minds work. They are not being nudged toward changing how they live their lives.

In sum, Gray's version of psychoanalysis includes a number of key features. He proposes a focus on the defensive action of the patient in an effort to help the patient understand the nature and sources of defensive activities as they have just occurred in the session. He recommends that the analyst's attention be directed to the patient's mind in session, not the patient's life outside the session. He argues against the effort to change the patient either through positive transference or through presenting a benign and approving stance toward the patient. Finally, since his focus is on helping patients observe themselves in session, he refrains from offering depth interpretations that point beyond what they can see. These elements of Gray's ego psychology point to a consistent stance toward the patient and to an interlocking set of analytic aims. Gray wants above all to enhance the patient's capacity for self-analysis and increase the ego's autonomy (1994, p. 26). Gray acknowledges the frankly educative component in helping patients become aware of their internal processes as they unfold in the session. To analyze a defense includes demonstrating its existence and motive to the analysand (p. 42). Gray wants to bring the rational aspects of the patient's ego on board (p. 48, footnote 8) in order to avoid irrational influences such as suggestion. He sees therapeutic change as one that is cognitive and experiential (p. 52). He refers to analysis as a scientific investigation that is shared by patient and analyst (p. 71). Both of them are coming to learn more about the patient's mind through a consideration of observable data, not through the intuitions of the analyst's unconscious attunement to the patient's unconscious. An effort is made to draw the patient's ego into conscious participation in the analytic process (p. 93). The ultimate aim is to assist the patient to "develop an increasingly autonomous capacity for an ever-freer intrapsychic spontaneity, reflectively observed and verbalized" (p. 61).

Gray seems to be proposing a number of valued outcomes for analysis that give shape to the kind of personhood or subjectivity that analysis can help people achieve: free intrapsychic spontaneity, increased autonomy, voluntary control over impulses, and rational capacity for reflective observation. When Gray critiques other psychoanalytic approaches he is usually doing so to protect one of these aims. Analysts of other schools can argue whether Gray's reasoned reflection on defense really enhances intrapsychic spontaneity. Do Gray's aims, laudable though they sound, obscure or interfere with the achievement of other aims that are also worthwhile, for example, the capacity for intimate attachments or liberated eros? Do his aims for analytic treatment rest upon a distorted picture of what is possible for people? Is there even something self-deceptive about the ideal of rational, self-reflective autonomy? Whether answers to these questions are supportive or critical of Gray will depend on the value accorded to the form of psychological life Gray is promoting. It is easy to see that this form of life is not the only one on offer in psychoanalysis by comparing it with that of other schools.

Bruce Fink's Lacanian Analysis

Any attempt to provide an overview of Bruce Fink's explication and interpretation of Lacanian psychoanalysis will encounter a number of difficulties. This is partly due to the well-known complexities of Lacanian theory. Any effort to spell out the theoretical underpinnings of and relationships between the concepts of need, demand, desire, satisfaction, object a, the fundamental fantasy (and its traversal), the subject's alienation in language, separation, the dialectization of desire, subjectification, etc. (let alone their implications for clinical practice) would require a book length effort. Or perhaps it would require several books, for Fink's work is just such an exposition carried out across multiple volumes.

But there is another reason why an overview of Fink's work is a troubled enterprise. There is an element of Lacanian thought that sets it in opposition to the effort to summarize. The effort to summarize is an effort to formulate and understand, and Lacan and Fink are decidedly "against understanding," to cite the title of Fink's two volumes of collected papers (Fink, 2014a, 2014b). One might object that the proscription on understanding is a matter of clinical practice in work with patients that does not apply to the attempt to explicate Fink's theoretical and clinical perspective on analysis. It is true that Fink's recommendations against understanding focus on clinical practice. But he also warns about the dangers in those efforts, including his own, which try to provide a theoretical summary of Lacanian thought. Fink writes of Lacan continually exploding "the emerging orthodox interpretations of his own teaching" (Fink, 1997, p. 218). This is not because Lacan always disapproves of the interpretations on offer.

> To Lacan's mind, a teaching worthy of the name must not end with the creation of a perfect, complete system; after all there is no such thing. A genuine teaching continues to evolve, to call itself into question, to forge new concepts.
>
> (Fink, 2004, p. 66)

It seems to me that a similar respect for the non-encapsulatable, multi-directional nature of Fink's own work is appropriate. Perhaps the best that can be done in a short exposition like this is to keep this idea of "the unfinished," "the not definitively formulatable" in mind as I go on to do some injustice to his work. As a first pass at a central theme of Fink's Lacanian analysis, one might understand the effort to be "unfixed" as pointing to a central aspect of Fink's notion of flourishing. There is something about the project to define oneself, or to surrender to another's comprehension of oneself, that undermines the particular version of flourishing that is promoted in this form of analysis.

In fact the patient's self-understanding constitutes one of the initial obstacles to doing analytic work. Patients come to treatment with any number of complaints and symptoms, and some ideas of what is wrong with them. They may approach analysis as the means to fix what they already "know" to be wrong with them, or to get the analyst's more professional take on what is wrong. But the analyst's job is to loosen patients' grip on what they know, not to offer alternative, "more accurate" knowledge about them. The aim is to help patients to begin to lose their grip on themselves, to become puzzled and curious about what they had previously assumed about themselves.[1] The dangers of a stultifying self-understanding that obscures the unconscious are not avoided by replacing the patient's view with the analyst's. The patient's self-understanding is itself an imposition from parents and the broader social world. The patient is already alienated and doesn't need a new alienation at the hands of the analyst, neither by adopting the analyst's ideas about them, nor by taking on the analyst's personal qualities. "The goal of analysis must *not* be identification with one's analyst, identification with the 'healthy part' of the analyst's ego, or identification with any other part of the analyst" (Fink, 1997, p. 63).

Hence, the analyst's interventions are not to be informative or interpersonally influential, but oracular. The analyst is not only trying to destabilize certain meanings and ideas that patients already have about themselves and their relationships, but also works to remain an allusive figure, someone who offers no firm set of ideas that patients can substitute for their own. The technique of punctuation is intended to do this. An emphatic "Huh!" or the repetition of a word or phrase that has multiple meanings beyond what the patient was intending to say points beyond what is conscious to an unconscious that may be slipping through in the patient's speech (see Fink, 1997, chapter 2, and 2007, chapter 3). Punctuation is usefully directed to any manifestations of the unconscious, which may be anything that interrupts speech, such as a slip of the tongue, breaking off a sentence half finished, mixed metaphors, pleonasms, retractions, etc. (see Fink, 2004, chapter 3). Scansion, the ending of a session at a moment of impactful manifestation of the unconscious, is a more emphatic punctuation that underlines what just happened in session and keeps the patient from covering it back over with a consciously "meaningful" discourse that undermines its force.

Interpretation as well should point to something in the analysand's speech in an enigmatic and polyvalent way that does not prescribe a set meaning for it. The aim is not to communicate a meaning but to have an impact, to promote the patient's curiosity about their unconscious, and to stimulate the patient's memories and associations. That is, the aim of techniques such as punctuation and interpretation is not simply negative, to break the hold of the patient's consciously intended self-understanding, but to produce in the patient's speech more of what had been previously avoided or repressed. Such techniques aim to set the patient to work following the trail of these pointers to the unconscious.

As an example of punctuation, Fink (2007, p. 92) describes repeating a phrase spoken by an analysand that had multiple meanings. This patient had spoken of his sense that he had not risen as high in a corporate hierarchy as he would expect at his age and complained of people trying to act as father figures toward him. The patient says, "I've often stumbled on my own ascent to power." Fink repeats the phrase "ascent to power," and the patient hears the ambiguity of "assent" alongside "ascent." This led to a shift in the patient's speech, not to what one might expect given the literal meaning of the alternative version of the phrase (i.e., not to the patient's sense of himself as assenting to power), but to his wishes to dominate others. This illustrates the principle that one cannot predict where such enigmatic interventions will take the patient, and that it is certainly not the goal to get the patient to see something the analyst already sees.

The analyst's interventions are intended to foster the patient's curiosity and interest in the unconscious and to provide a place in the patient's speech for the unconscious to make its ambiguous appearance. The analyst is guided by what can be discerned of the patient's unconscious appearing alongside any consciously intended meanings, not by the hunt for themes generated by psychoanalytic theory (oedipal themes, sibling rivalry, etc.). Nevertheless, Fink does think that there are specifics about patients the analyst ought to inquire about. It is possible for patients to drone on endlessly about day-to-day events that have little significance. There are aspects of patients' lives that are more likely to be relevant to analytic process and to patients' psychodynamics. The details of patients' family structures and histories; of their childhood experiences; and of their dreams, fantasies, and sexual experiences need to be actively elicited. The analyst does not just wait for patients to get around to such topics.

Details matter about almost any topic the patient brings up. Analysts are never to assume that they understand what a patient has said based on experiences of their own, or on some sense of what "anyone" would feel in a particular situation. The focus on the particulars of this patient's life should never be abandoned. When a patient reports that they were fired, got a promotion, broke up with a girlfriend, or heard that their sister's husband has cancer, one shouldn't assume they felt frightened, angry, sad, or jubilant, or that one knows the meanings of those events. One has to get the patient talking about them.

Fink is wary about analysts who set themselves up as having specialized knowledge to give their patients. This has implications for how to handle transference as well. Telling the patient that their perception of or reaction to the analyst is transference, or interpreting whence it comes ("You're seeing me as a pompous authority figure just as you've always seen your father") does not change transference. The patient will simply hear the interpretation from within the same perspective ("That's just like my father—telling me what I'm 'really' up to"). Further, it points patients in the wrong direction, toward whether or not they are accurately perceiving the analyst. The analyst is not where the patient needs to look. Transference needs to be investigated as to its source, not its accuracy.

Consider the following exchange. A patient has been talking wearily and dejectedly about his parents for several sessions, initially emphasizing that his mother seemed like an obstacle to anyone enjoying themselves. He spoke of her being afraid of everything, how she imposed her fears on others, setting limits on what she would allow family members to do—and on how much money could be spent in doing it, for one of her greatest fears concerned family finances. But in this session the patient begins to speak of the sharp edge in some of his father's comments about the patient's mother.

Patient: "Dad would complain about mom's 'economizing' as though she were stealing all his fun."

Analyst: "You put air quotes around 'economizing.'"

Patient: "Are you saying she really was cheap?! No quotes needed? (Long exhale.) God, it pissed me off when Dad would speak sarcastically about mom economizing when he just meant she was cheap and stingy. I hated it when he did that, made those sarcastic put downs—but I also felt I was supposed to agree with him, and I guess I sort of did. I thought you were putting her down, too, when you said that, that I shouldn't mince words, I should just call her cheap."

Analyst: "You hated your father putting your mother down."

Patient: "Yeah, like an old dog."

Analyst: "Putting her down like an old dog."

The patient hears the reference to euthanizing and goes on to talk of a time when there was a possibility that his mother had cancer, and the "strange feeling" he had that his father would not have been unhappy if she did have cancer and died. This led to remembering his own fantasies at the time of what it would be like if she died: "Weird. I just had an image of my childhood home filled with light. What the hell is that?!"

In this example, the analyst does not take up the question of whether the patient misunderstood the analyst, or was seeing the analyst as sarcastically critical like his father, or whether the patient was angry with both father and analyst for implying what the patient thought himself (that his mother was cheap). Instead, transference is understood as a derailing of the associative process. The patient is brought back into this process, his strong affect regarding his father is underlined, an unintended meaning of "putting someone down" is noted, and further links to childhood memories result. The aim of work with transference is to follow associative links to its origins in childhood and infancy, not to point out to the patient that it is being enacted with the analyst.

Fink aims at an analysis that seeks to break up patients' fixed ideas about themselves in order to set in motion a curiosity about the unconscious and an attunement to its manifestations in their speech. To what end? Is this just about curiosity and following the tell-tale signs of the unconscious for its own sake? No, for there is fixation not simply at the level of the ego's "self-knowledge" (which isn't genuine, since the ego that would understand itself is always fundamentally deluded; see Fink, 2004, p. 45). There is also a fixation of desire. Patients have been erotically fixated, repeating the same patterns of interaction with others, positioning themselves in ways that repeat a truncated or stunted enjoyment in life, unable to pursue satisfaction more directly. The patient feels obliged to enact a certain position or stance in life. This position keeps the patient in orbit, circling around a real satisfaction without allowing the patient to approach it. The aim of analysis is to free the patient from this fixation, to no longer live a form of life imposed from without and unconsciously taken up by the patient. Such fixations lead patients to frustrating entrapment in agendas that are fundamentally dead ends: to constantly try to expose authority figures' hypocrisy (as revenge on a pompous father); to compensate parents for a sibling's death; to have the exciting sex life that mother never had; to assuage a father's sense of failure by being successful; to prove that mom was wrong to idealize a sibling, etc.

To be freed from such fixations is to be freed to make one's life one's own. This is not the freedom to choose a life the way one chooses which shoes to buy. This choosing is not the act of an absolute sovereign, but there is still a kind of ownership or "subjectification." This is perhaps a psychoanalytic version of Nietzsche's "yes-saying," an affirmation of a life that is given, and that operates in stark contrast to the superego's "No!"

Furthering the analysand's Eros is the aim of psychoanalysis (Fink, 1995, p. 146). This doesn't mean that the patient becomes a "non-stop pleasure-seeking machine" (Fink, 1997, p. 210), but that the patient no longer repeatedly enacts alienating desires in a way that interferes with their satisfaction. In the process, other things will change in ways that match the standard aims of other analytic schools and of other therapies. Fink (2017, p. 285) writes of his analysands "having more energy, being less plagued by fantasies they find repulsive, being able to stand up for themselves, finally feeling they have a voice of their own, etc." These are effects of the analytic process, but they are not directly aimed at by that process.

A further outcome returns us to our beginning point. When Fink writes (for example, in 1997, chapter 10) of the shift in the later Lacan from a focus on desire to one on drive, he notes that Lacan had come to see that only drive can make it possible to get out from under the dominance of expectations internalized from the Other (from parents and the larger social world) that have shaped the patient's desires. Fink frames this shift in Lacan's later theory not so much as a change in the fundamental aims of analysis, but as a change in how those aims are conceptualized. "The goal remains to separate from the Other, and to enable the subject to pursue his or her course without all the inhibitions and influences that derive from concrete others around the subject or the internalized Other's values and judgments" (Fink, 1997, p. 207). Fink sees this goal as consonant with the general thrust of Lacan's work, from early to late. It is also central to Fink's characterization of analysis as "non-normalizing," as eschewing the many tendencies to generate norms for development, reality testing, and proper functioning out of a universal theory of human nature (see 2007, chapter 9). Rather than being moved toward conformity with standard norms,

> by the end of their analyses, analyzed people are probably some of the most 'abnormal' people around! They tend to follow their own bents, caring little about fitting into molds, and are slave to neither social conventions nor the flouting of such conventions.
>
> (Fink, 2017, p. 325)

So the danger noted at the beginning, that of doing an injustice to Fink's work in summarizing it, parallels the injustice (alienation) done to analysands by virtue of being part of a social/symbolic/linguistic world. It is the aim of psychoanalysis to address the effect on the analysand of alienating social molds imposed upon and accepted by the analysand. Psychoanalysis is a project of liberation from the impositions of the Other.

The liberation from familial and social conformity for the sake of the libidinal vitality of the drives is a very different sort of aim from the increased autonomy sought in Gray's analysis. Fink's aim is not Gray's, not a strengthened ego that has overcome irrational defenses against instinctual impulses and instituted a practice of reasoned decision about when and how to give expression to them. From Fink's perspective the educative aspect of Gray's practice is a setup for alienation, not autonomy. The analysand can quickly discern what the ego psychologist's intentions are (to develop a capacity for rational reflection on defensive processes) and begin to try to be a good student, to be someone who acts in service to this aim of the analyst. For Fink, analysis aims at throwing off the constrictions of others' expectations (and of the search for someone to provide such expectations) in order to be freed up to let the drive be one's own, to follow it without any assessment of its worth or reasonableness against an external standard. This sounds like it would put Fink in direct conflict with Charles Taylor on the centrality of strong evaluation. However, to be liberated from externally imposed standards is not to pursue something simply because one happens to want it (i.e., it is not an example of weak evaluation). Liberation from the impositions of Others is clearly an ideal, even if Fink's version of this is not something one can turn into a deliberate project.

Stephen Mitchell's Relational Analysis

Throughout his writings Stephen Mitchell repeatedly turns to other psychoanalytic theorists to provide a context for his own views. This is true not only of his books that are expressly written to survey the history of analytic thought, such as *Object Relations in Psychoanalytic Theory* (Greenberg & Mitchell, 1983) or *Freud and Beyond* (Mitchell & Black, 1995). Consider, for example, a chapter on the analyst's intentions in *Influence and Autonomy in Psychoanalysis* (Mitchell, 1997). He begins with pointed questions about "what we should be trying to do" as analysts. He then presents one of his cases. Eventually he uses this case to illustrate what he thinks the analyst's intentions should be—but not before considering over the next twenty-four pages a number of theorists' ideas about their intentions to be neutral (Sigmund Freud, Kernberg, Anna Freud), or empathic (Kohut), or containing (Bion) or holding (Winnicott). Mitchell presents what he thinks by locating himself in relation to what others have to say.

Certainly, providing the historical context or justification for new psychoanalytic ideas is characteristic of much analytic writing. But it is not always so prominent or pervasive a part of theoretical exposition or technical recommendations. It is not so central to Gray and Fink, for example. Fink's work is largely a commentary on and clinical elaboration of Lacan's work, with occasional asides on other analysts. Gray writes about Sigmund Freud and Anna Freud as laying the foundations for his own position. He contrasts his approach to analysis with that of others (Kohut, for example), but he does not lay the groundwork for his views with a detailed consideration of the broad range of past and present analytic theorizing. Mitchell does. On his way to a theory of psychoanalysis as a relational practice Mitchell is relational in his practice of theorizing.

Mitchell's continual return to the history of theory could be a function of his role as an educator. It may also be what he felt he needed to do rhetorically to gain acceptance for an approach to psychoanalysis that was likely to be perceived by some as jettisoning essential aspects of psychoanalysis, like drive theory and technical neutrality. Perhaps a review of history presented a sort of advance defense: "Don't accuse me of blindly throwing out the baby with the bathwater—I have well-reasoned ideas based on careful consideration of opposing views as to which is the baby and which is the bathwater."

But I think it is just as plausible that he is practicing a relational approach to theorizing as a complement to his relational theory of analysis, a theory whose central idea is that we are what and who we are in and through our relationships with others. Further, Mitchell doesn't seem to think this is an unusual approach to theorizing.

> No psychoanalytic theorist builds theory just to express his own thought or to share her clinical findings. Each also selects from the by-now enormous and heterogeneous collections of psychoanalytic perspectives

some particular points of reference, with the intent to expand and develop some and to contrast with and argue with others.

(Mitchell, 1993, p. 157)

But few theorists do this expanding, contrasting, and arguing as thoroughly as Mitchell does.

Mitchell's examinations of other psychoanalytic theories and clinical practices are not neutral. He lays them out not simply to categorize them into those he is closer to or further from. His intent is polemical. He is building a case for a relational psychoanalysis as more plausible than a drive theory like Freud's or "developmental arrest theories" (as he calls them) like Winnicott's and Kohut's. He does not think it is tenable to subscribe to important ideas from the history of analysis as though they were universally true, *the* touchstone for theory and practice. Nevertheless, he is not out to abandon as clinically useless the theories he critiques. He acknowledges the potential relevance of Oedipal dynamics in the neurotic; of patterns of love, hate, envy, and reparations in early childhood; or of injuries to patients stemming from impingement or failures of attunement in the past. The history of psychoanalysis provides the analyst with a wealth of material that can be useful in illuminating the dynamics of particular patients. "Basic concepts within psychoanalytic theory provide interpretive possibilities for orienting the clinician toward crucial and hidden dimensions of meaning by informing his sensibilities as a listener" (Greenberg & Mitchell, 1983, pp. 15–16). Mitchell believes that one has to make a choice between fundamental models such as drive theory or relational theory. But a particular patient's relational dynamics may take on forms that were first spelled out in any number of specific traditional theories (Freudian Oedipal competition, Kleinian envious spoiling, Kohutian idealizing, etc.). Such specific relational configurations are not, however, to be used as favored templates to be laid over whatever any patient presents. The analyst needs to listen to (and, as we shall see, be pulled into) the particular dynamics of a given patient in order to discover what those dynamics are—and they may not neatly fit any of the standard patterns.

In explicating the relational model, Mitchell finds the clearest contrasting perspective to be Freud's drive theory. He characterizes Freud as proposing a picture of people as having biologically based drives of a sexual and aggressive nature that necessarily put them in conflict with the social world. Such drives are what is most fundamental about being human, and they put people at odds with societal efforts to contain and control the expression of those sexual and aggressive wishes. By contrast,

the relational model rests on the premise that the repetitive patterns within human experience are not derived, as in the drive model, from pursuing gratification of inherent pressures and pleasures ... but from a pervasive tendency to preserve the continuity, connections, familiarity of one's personal, interactional world.

(Mitchell, 1988, p. 33)

Mitchell is not denying that people can behave and experience themselves as driven, or as sexually and aggressively "bestial," or as demandingly self-centered. But he does not see this as evidence of the operation of drives or the vestiges of a primary narcissism. Rather, such ways of living (and of understanding oneself) are reified patterns of relating to others that arose in the particular interpersonal contexts of an individual's relationship history.

Further, the chief concern of analysis is not to replace the patient's templates of interpersonal life with "better" ones, nor to correct what is false in a patient's self-understanding. Rather, the problem is that relational patterns and their corresponding sense of self have become reified and fixed. With regard to sexual patterns, for example, it is not the content but the rigidity of the pattern that is most often problematic. This is true for sexual relationships that are often labeled as perverse (sadism, masochism, fetishism). But rigidity or fixity of sexual relationships is also at the heart of problems in other sexual scenarios. For example, it is not the particular act but the compulsive repetition that is the problem Mitchell (1988, p. 116) sees in the case of a woman who flirted with other men in order to get revenge on her husband for his lack of sexual interest in her. Relational patterns in sexual relationships become pathological when they are stereotyped and compulsive rather than open to "various relational themes characterized by both mutual discovery and mutual defiance, where meanings pertaining to search and accommodation, and rebellion (both against each other and, jointly, against social norms) find a place within the same sequence of actions" (Mitchell, 1988, p. 118).

Mitchell is also critical of developmental arrest theories. He sees aspects of Winnicott's and Kohut's theories, for example, as painting a picture of psychopathology as a sort of "deficiency disease" (Mitchell, 1988, p. 130). Such theories propose that early in life the patient was not provided with what everyone needs (appropriate holding, or non-impinging attunement, or mirroring, or opportunities for symbiotic merger or idealization, etc.). The analyst's job is to replace the missing parental function. The implication of such a model is that if the child were given the proper provisions there would be no problems and life would be free of frustration, stunted development, and conflict. Mitchell does not accept this picture of psychological problems as the direct result of deprivations. He sees the child as an active participant in creating an interpersonal world out of whatever is available to them. This was true in childhood when these patterns were created, and it is also true of adults: we are "active creators and loyal perpetuators of conflictual relational patterns" (Mitchell, 1988, p. 172). Indeed, the relational crucible in which such patterns are formed is inevitably conflictual. There is no relationship between mother and child (or father and child, or sibling and child, etc.) that is free of conflict, frustration, and disappointment. Mitchell sometimes calls his approach to analysis a "relational-conflict model." Hence, the analyst's job is not to provide what the patient was previously deprived of, but to lead them to relinquish ties to old patterns.

How? Not simply by pointing out these patterns to the patient, although that may certainly happen along the way. Indeed, for Mitchell, providing patients knowledge about themselves is hardly the central mode of therapeutic action. In fact, the patient may be *less* known at the end of analytic treatment than at the beginning (Mitchell, 1993, p. 121). Mitchell contrasts his approach with the classical Freudian model of therapeutic process. The aim of the latter could be put under the heading of "know thyself." Freud takes as his model of healthy maturity the sober scientist unflinchingly facing personal truths, however unsavory. According to Mitchell, for much of contemporary analysis, including his own relational model, the aim is closer to "express thyself" (where the artist is the model of psychological health, not the scientist; see Mitchell, 2002, p. 109).

So what do psychoanalytic interventions do? How do they help the patient relinquish ties to old relational patterns? Consider the quintessential analytic intervention, interpretation.

> In the classical model … the information conveyed by the interpretation reveals hidden content, lifts repression barriers, and thereby shifts the internal balance of psychic forces. In the developmental-arrest model, the interpretation has its effect in the *experience* it generates in the patient, who feels deeply cared about and understood … In the relational-conflict model, both the informational content and affective tone are regarded as crucial, but their effects are understood somewhat differently … An interpretation … says something very important about where the analyst stands vis-à-vis the analysand, about what sort of relatedness is possible between them.
>
> (Mitchell, 1988, pp. 294–295)

The interpretation doesn't just convey information, but enacts a different sort of relatedness than had previously existed between patient and analyst.

Mitchell holds that the analyst is inevitably drawn into a sort of countertransference position with the patient that repeats (in some sense) that patient's prior relational patterns. The analyst's job is to pay attention to this happening, and engage the patient in collaborative investigation into how the two of them got there. An interpretation that addresses this relational re-enactment aims to place the two of them into this position of collaborative inquiry. But it also aims to open a space for a different relational alternative to a patient's previous patterns. These are not restitutions, not the provision of the "good" relationship the patient never had, but alternatives that free the patient from constricting relational patterns. Because the relational patterns that people bring to analysis can be so various, the helpful alternative relational positionings of the analyst will be just as various. There are no general rules for how to do this. So Mitchell is critical of the notion that there is a default position the analyst should adopt, even if one adds the option for modifications depending on the patient's needs or level of pathology. One cannot say that the fundamental analytic stance is neutrality, empathy, abstinence, holding, mirroring, anonymity, etc. Whatever position analysts think they are adopting in relation to their patients may simply be experienced by patients through the lens of their old patterns (Mitchell refers to this as the "bootstrapping problem"; see Mitchell, 1997, pp. 44–53). Analysts may think they are being neutral, but their patients may experience them as cold. Analysts may think they are being empathic, but their patients may see them as pitying or condescending. Rather than a generically ideal position that is valid for any analysis, the position the analyst seeks should be one that provides an alternative to the positions in which the patient typically places others, including the analyst. Such an alternative will in turn alter the correlative position of the patient.

With no single analytic position to be adopted, and no fundamental technique held up as the core analytic intervention, it is difficult to extract from Mitchell a simple picture of his recommendations for practice. Because his work is formed in the context of the particular relational dynamics of specific patients the significance of a given intervention or interpretation can be seen only by placing it in that context.

Consider his case of Rachel (Mitchell, 1997, pp. 170–175 and 199–201). He describes a young woman who had been living in a sort of passive fog with a boyfriend whom she described as spending his days smoking marijuana, watching television, and playing video games. When treatment began she had her own ethereal, marijuana-magnified spaciness. This gradually dissipated as she became more vibrant, quit frequent pot smoking, and entered graduate school. After completing a master's degree, she was contemplating applying to a doctoral program, but Mitchell began to see elements of self-sabotage in how she was delaying the completion of her application, as though she were now neglecting herself the way her parents had when she applied to undergraduate programs. Mitchell notes that at this time he was dealing with his own daughter's applications to New York City high schools, a process in which he was actively engaged.

At this point in treatment Mitchell began to feel a sense of urgency about Rachel, that she may have been undermining her options. But he also questioned this sense of urgency. Was he feeling a competitive urge to be a better parent than her parents? "Was I being seduced into being a rescuing father? Was I seducing her into being a neglected daughter in need of rescue?" (Mitchell, 1997, p. 174). Was the urgency he felt a sign he was about to misstep into an enactment and should remain silent? Or would silence have been a repetition of her parents' failure to be involved?

He raised these and other questions in his private reflections on the treatment. What he ended up doing was describing the position he saw her occupying, and how he found himself responding to it:

> You know, it is my impression from talking to you and listening to what you say about other people's responses to you, that you are an extremely talented woman. Because you so expect a lack of positive response, you play it safe by setting things up to make it unlikely that you will get where you want to go. I think your parents really neglected you by not helping you with the college applications and that you are in danger of repeating that neglect yourself by not being more active now. I am aware of having the impulse to ask you to bring in the applications so that I can go over them with you. I am not sure whether actually doing that would be a good thing or a bad thing, helpful or not, but I wanted to tell you what I was thinking.
>
> (Mitchell, 1997, p. 200)

What was important was talking with her about not only what he saw her doing with the application, but how that affected him, so they both could look at the interpersonal dynamics that were being played out between them. Rachel had a strong response to what Mitchell said at the moment. In the next session she told him she thought he was right about what she had been doing in delaying the applications. She didn't ask him to help her to do them, and noted that she found it scary to take herself seriously. In his comment to her, Mitchell offered her an invitation to look at herself differently, as he took her seriously, while sharing with her how he was affected by her.

In being so direct with Rachel about his experience of her, wasn't there a risk that he would be pushing her to be how he thought she should be? Perhaps. But is it realistic to assume that one can hide the patient's impact on the analyst, and the analyst's reaction to that impact? Mitchell does not believe it is wise to try to hide the influence of patient and analyst on each other in order to protect the patient's autonomy from the analyst's influence.

> The most constructive safeguard of the autonomy of the patient is not the denial of the personal impact of the analyst but the acknowledgment,

both in our theoretical concepts and in our clinical work, of the interactive nature of the analytic process.

(Mitchell, 1997, p. 28)

Further, even if Rachel does internalize something from Mitchell, this is not necessarily self-alienating. Mitchell borrows from Loewald the contrast between repression and internalization, where the former is the ego's defensive action that results in closing oneself off to something in oneself, and the latter involves the ego's opening itself up to the world (Mitchell, 2000, p. 43). Opening up is not necessarily submission, but may be engagement.

Because each patient's relational dynamics are different, one cannot draw up general rules for how to listen and respond. "*What* one does is less important than how openly what does happen is *processed* with the analysand" (Mitchell, 1997, p. x). One will inevitably be drawn into a particular sort of relationship with each patient, a relationship shaped by the patient's recurring patterns, but also by the ways the particular analyst, with their own personal history, shaped by their analytic training and theoretical predilections, is able to be shaped. The analyst's work is to listen to and observe the patient, but also to sense or feel the relational pulls and configurations that arise. Who is this person being with me? Who do I find myself being with the patient? Why am I so cautious? Am I afraid of something? Do I see the patient as fragile, feel that I must tread lightly? Does the patient somehow help to create this picture of fragility as a warning to me? To avoid something else? Does the patient fear being "too much" for me? Does this say something (maybe more) about me than about the patient, something I am afraid of about myself?

Analysts will have a preliminary glimpse of a relationship forming and re-forming between themselves and their patients, and part of the work is to explore the relationships' contours, demands, traps, etc. Eventually, analysts engage their patients in joint consideration of how they arrived at this particular relational configuration. This is not a matter of a continual running commentary on the relationship between analyst and analysand. Many, even most sessions may have no direct comment or inquiry on the state of the relationship. But the relationship is ultimately where the therapeutic action is. It is only through patient and analyst being pulled into a particular sort of relationship with each other that the heart of the patient's relational patterns are revealed in a live way. In this respect, Mitchell's take on the centrality of transference is not markedly different from views held by many analysts, including Freud. But Mitchell does not think this re-animation of transferential/relational patterns is simply the distorting influence of the past on a current "real relationship" that the analyst can observe accurately from outside the distortion. Such patterns do start in and have something to do with past relationships and an exploration of that may be helpful. But such relational patterns are not hold-overs that are inappropriate to the present. They create the present in a form that is familiar from the past. The present relationship is being lived by both participants in ways the patient knows, is familiar with, feels safe with, and uses for certain purposes to address certain problems, needs, or wishes. And, of course, these ways of being in relationship also create problems.

How do analysts formulate, for themselves and their patients, what they sense is happening between them? A variety of psychoanalytic theories can be helpful as guideposts in this task. Analysts' knowledge of Oedipal dynamics, schizoid and depressive positions, empathic needs, etc. gives them a set of narratives regarding types of relational configurations that can appear, while remaining alert to the possibility that a particular patient's dynamic may not fit neatly into any such framework.

The psychoanalytic tradition also points to particular sorts of experiences that form the setting in which relational patterns are first formed: separations and losses, overstimulation, physical pain and illness, glimpses of mortality, exclusion from the parental relationship, sibling comparison and competition, dependency, etc. (see Mitchell, 1988, p. 276).

By opening a conversation with Rachel about what he saw her doing with herself, in relationship to him, and how he found himself wanting to respond (to rescue her), Mitchell creates a space in which they can look anew at what is happening. It allows both of them to step back—Mitchell from the urge to rescue, Rachel from her dismissive inattention to her ambitions, talents, and wishes. Is this so that they can go on to the "correct relationship" of Rachel to herself, and of each to the other? There is an idea that something beneficial has happened here, that Mitchell has regained his analytic footing so that he can talk with her about what is going on. Similarly, implicit in the intervention is the idea that it is better for Rachel to take herself seriously. But there is no suggestion that this will be *the* form of what either of them consider better for analytic work or Rachel's life. The further unfolding of analysis may take them both through further transformations regarding where to find the better engagement with each other or with broader life choices.

The aim here then is not a particular better analytic relationship or positioning of Rachel toward herself, but to learn to engage in a process of exploration of what is happening with oneself in relation to another. The process is not intended to arrive at fixed conclusions, but to develop a curiosity that loosens rigid patterns that have been compulsively and unconsciously lived out. The aim is an openness to the complexity, ambiguity, and depth of human experience in relationship.

Divergent Psychoanalytic Aims

Mitchell's relational analysis aims at an appreciation of the complexity of persons in relationship, the fostering of a habit of curiosity, a willingness to re-find oneself as other than one thought one was, differently positioned than one had been before. Mitchell applauds patients' searches for personal meaning in analysis, and would accept that some meanings are better than others (i.e., they resolve certain problems or provide paths out of particular dead ends). But the more fundamental aim is to be open to the search, which entails that no meanings are final or unambiguous. Finding the best meaning is less important than a sustained curiosity about meaning. In a sense, Mitchell shares Fink's concerns about fixing "who one is" in a formula of self-understanding. But for Mitchell, having *some* self-understanding, making sense of who one is, is inevitable and is not simply alienating. Fink might agree that to be a person is to be in relation to others, and that to be this person rather than that one is partly constituted by how I place myself vis-à-vis others (via a fundamental fantasy). But Mitchell emphasizes that our influence on each other is not only unavoidable, but provides one of the central arenas within which analysts can help to free someone from previous deleterious influence. The troubles that arise in the interpersonal field can most fruitfully be addressed interpersonally. The aim is to free people from interpersonal traps in order to enrich the relational world in which they inevitably live.

Fink, of course, could concede that relational influence is always present, but that it is not what psychoanalysis is about, nor the medium of its effects. In fact, he would consider it that from which patients need to be freed. On this score, he and Gray might agree (whatever else they would disagree about). However, Gray might question the validity of Lacanian ideas about freeing the unconscious, setting people free from how others have shaped them (and from their own participation in this alienation), by following the derailments and ambiguities of speech. He would claim there is a much more experience-near path for patients to follow in freeing up the repressed. Patients can become skilled at the detection and dismantling of defense and take over the analytic process set in motion with the analyst's aid. Mitchell would agree with Gray that analysis is ultimately a collaborative enterprise, although for Mitchell this is less of a learned skill than joint reflection following joint participation in a relational experience. For Fink, too, the patient is hardly the passive recipient of analytic intervention. Interpretation and punctuation are intended to set the analysand to work, following the trail of the unconscious revealed in speech and symptom. But this does not give patients more knowledge about themselves regarding either their defenses or their relational patterns. Instead, it destabilizes such "knowledge." There is no joint project here to articulate with the patient what the patient has been doing defensively or relationally in order to find a way to do things differently. There is simply the undoing of imaginary self-understandings and of alienating, repetitive desires in order to free patients to pursue their satisfaction—what that is or where that might take the patient is not the business of analysis.

How are we to understand the differences between these approaches to psychoanalysis? They are at least in part explained by competing notions of flourishing, of what makes a life full or worthwhile. Each of these forms of analysis focuses on a different aim: the capacity to reflect on and alter defense; liberation from narcissistic self-constructions and fixated trajectories of desire; curiosity about and reflection on shifting interpersonal patterns.

What would it mean to say that one school of analysis has it "right," or at least more right than another? Would it be to say that that school sees what is most fundamental to psychological dynamics and motivations, or to subjectivity as linguistically constituted? Don't the practices of these different analyses in fact focus on patients (and/or their relationship to the analyst) in such a way as to highlight that in the analysand which supports the tenets of the theory? And by ushering the patient through these practices, don't they help to create what they are about, to discover/create and then reconfigure, change, or liberate the patient from the defenses, relational patterns, and alienating self-concepts and desires that these analytic theories posit as the central focus of analytic work? Don't they, in a sense, "make themselves true," to borrow a phrase from the philosopher Alasdair MacIntyre (1985)?

If therapeutic theories create what they find (or if the distinction between creation and discovery is necessarily blurred here) this is not because they create the problems they address out of whole cloth, as though people were blank slates upon which different analysts write whatever they want. People bring something specific to analysis, but what they bring is given new form in the context of these distinct analytic "environments." Different analytic theories and practices include distinct ideas about the nature of persons, about what is beneficial and harmful to them.

What is damaging or limiting and what is good in this context are not simply observed the way one observes medical illness (a wound, a limp), or physical health (the robust stride of a strong runner). Or, to the extent that they are observable (the downcast face and posture of depression, the restless agitation of anxiety, the intense vigilant stare of paranoia), they are explicated through particular therapeutic ideas about what matters in life, how flourishing is derailed, and what can make life better. Such ideas can be argued for and contested, illustrated with clinical narratives and personal testimony, supported by suggestive links to research findings from psychology and other disciplines in the social and biological sciences. But the possibility of definitive conclusions here is as likely as it is in politics. Does this mean anything goes, or that argumentation about flourishing is just an empty effort at persuasion that masquerades as reasoning? Certainly, such argumentation does not look like ordinary empirical research. There is no objective measure to appeal to in weighing one picture of flourishing against another. Debates about such matters are wide ranging, come in multiple forms, and entail appeals to basic ethical intuitions shared by the participants. They are fundamentally difficult, ambiguous, and never finished. As a consequence they are often ignored or assumed to be resolved through a loyalty to one's own perspective that dispenses with consideration of the alternatives. I am pointing to the presence of such ethical disagreements in therapy in order to suggest that these debates deserve closer consideration. In the companion volume *Therapeutic Ethics in Context and in Dialogue* I examine more closely what it means to directly engage in conversation about alternative visions of well-being.

However, some might contend that these disputes are not just resistant to resolution, but irrelevant. Do the different ethics of different therapies matter if we can establish that some therapies simply work better than others? I turn to this question in Chapter 5.

Note

1 I am focusing here on Fink's recommendations for working with neurotic patients.

5   Psychotherapy Research

From Effective Techniques to Ethical Aspirations

In the preceding two chapters I examined different therapies in order to illustrate how they promote different visions of human well-being. However, from an empirical perspective on therapy one might question whether differences in ethical vision matter. If one type of therapy works better than another, why should we care about its underlying view of flourishing? To put it simply, if depressed patients in cognitive-behavioral therapy are less likely to commit suicide than those in psychodynamic or humanistic therapy, then isn't that sufficient evidence that it more thoroughly improves well-being, regardless of any differences in underlying ethics between these schools of therapy? We know that, other things being equal, people suffering from severe symptoms of anxiety or depression are not living well. Wouldn't evidence that one form of therapy works better than another to reduce those symptoms be all we need to show that it was more successful at enhancing well-being? This is clearly part of the rationale for the project to identify evidence-based treatments (American Psychological Association Division 12 Task Force, 1995; Chambless & Hollon, 1998; Nathan & Gorman, 1998; Tolin et al., 2015).

Correlatively, if there is little evidence that therapy of one orientation is consistently more efficacious than another, this makes the exploration of differences in therapeutic ethics more significant. If different therapies are equivalently effective in symptom reduction, then allegiance to one therapy over another is better explained by the appeal of its picture of human flourishing.

There are those who argue that psychotherapy research is too flawed to give it much weight in comparative assessment of the therapies. Clinicians often raise objections to the research, questioning the relevance for practice of claims such as "Research has proven that therapy A is the most efficacious treatment for disorder X." Most clinicians see patients who have complex presentations, meet criteria for multiple disorders, or have complications that make it impractical to routinely apply a packaged treatment to a particular disorder. But researchers also have doubts about the data. Parker and Fletcher

(2007) and Shedler (2018) argue that the evidence to warrant the designation "empirically supported therapy" is far weaker than is routinely claimed, especially for the short-term manualized therapies that are typically so named. Cuijpers et al. (2010) argue that publication bias has generally inflated the estimate of effect sizes for various treatments. Ioannidis (2005) and researchers participating in Open Science Collaboration (2012) have raised doubts about the accuracy and reproducibility of much of the existing biomedical and psychological research.[1]

I have sympathy for such critiques, and they suggest that some of the findings presented in the text that follows should be taken with a grain of salt. Nevertheless, it seems foolish to ignore psychotherapy research findings that provide at least some attempt to go beyond the anecdotal and polemical views of proponents and critics of therapy. Further, if the research is weak it provides less reason to promote one therapy above another on the basis of its efficacy and more reason to consider that what differentiates the therapies are their distinct visions of living well.

Research on Differential Therapeutic Efficacy

While most research shows that therapy is generally efficacious (Lambert, 2013), there has been recurring controversy surrounding the question of whether some therapies work better than others. Eysenck (1966) found that therapies based on learning theory were more effective than psychoanalytic or eclectic therapies. Meltzoff and Kornreich (1970) found no evidence for the superiority of one type of treatment over another. Luborsky et al. (1975) agreed with Meltzoff and Kornreich on their general conclusion, with a caveat on the superiority of behavioral treatment for circumscribed phobias.

These early literature reviews were vulnerable to a number of biases that made it difficult to interpret their conclusions. The results of meta-analyses tend to support the view that the psychotherapies are generally equivalent in efficacy. Smith et al. (1980) concluded: "Different types of psychotherapy (verbal or behavioral; psychodynamic, client-centered, or systematic desensitization) do not produce different types or degrees of benefit" (p. 184). More recent meta-analytic studies have reached similar conclusions. Wampold et al. (1997) studied 277 comparisons of psychotherapies. The preponderance of the studies yielded little to no difference between therapies. The number of studies that yielded a larger difference between treatments was close to what one would expect by chance. Further, comparisons between treatments that were quite different (e.g., cognitive-behavioral vs. humanistic psychotherapy) showed no greater difference in efficacy than studies that compared two therapies of the same type (two cognitive-behavioral therapies).

However, general comparative research examining whether one type of therapy works better than another is not particularly illuminating. Medical researchers don't ask whether aspirin works better than an antibiotic. They ask whether one treatment works better than another for a particular condition or disease. Some meta-analyses have examined the effectiveness of specific psychotherapies for specific mental disorders. Wampold and Imel (2015) reviewed the evidence regarding differential efficacy for specific disorders (depression, anxiety disorders, and alcohol abuse). They found few differences between therapies for the treatment of specific disorders, with a few exceptions. Some meta-analyses they reviewed did find a superiority of cognitive-behavioral therapy for depression over other psychotherapies. However, many of the treatments that were compared to cognitive-behavioral therapy were not bona fide therapies. That is, the non-cognitive-behavioral therapy in many of these studies did not have a clear rationale, the therapists were not skilled practitioners, or they were artificially restricted in how they practiced the alternative therapy. These limitations reduced the efficacy of the comparison therapies and cast doubt on the conclusion that cognitive-behavioral therapy was more effective.

The bias that results from comparing bona fide treatments to spurious ones is related to problems that arise from the therapeutic allegiance of researchers. Research has identified the bias that results when the researcher conducting a study comparing the efficacy of two treatments has an allegiance to one of them. When meta-analyses of such comparisons control for allegiance, the difference between treatments is negligible (Luborsky et al., 1999; Munder et al., 2013).

It would be misleading to suggest that all research points to equivalence of therapies. One possible area of differential efficacy of treatments for depression can be found if one looks at targeted variables or disorder-specific symptom measures. That is, scores on symptom self-reports (such as the Beck Depression Inventory) show a small difference between cognitive-behavioral therapy and other therapies in the treatment of depression (see Tolin, 2010). Tolin found an even larger difference between cognitive-behavioral therapy and other therapies in the treatment of anxiety. However, Baardseth et al. (2013) challenged Tolin's conclusions, noting problems with the selection of studies for inclusion in his meta-analysis, the value of considering measures that are not disorder specific, and the fact that several other meta-analyses yield very different conclusions (see also Steinert et al., 2017; and the response to Baardseth et al. in Tolin, 2014).

The superiority of behavioral, cognitive-behavioral, and exposure-based therapies for various anxiety disorders is often cited in the literature (Nathan & Gorman, 1998; Roth & Fonagy, 2005), even by those who find little difference between treatments more generally (e.g., Frank & Frank, 1991).

Lambert et al. (2016) reach a similar conclusion in their overview of research on humanistic therapies. While humanistic therapies are generally equivalent in efficacy to other types of treatment, the research shows a small but significant advantage to cognitive-behavioral therapy in the treatment of some anxiety disorders. Wampold and colleagues (Benish et al., 2008; Wampold & Imel, 2015) have challenged this idea, arguing that claims for the superiority of these treatments is often exaggerated beyond what the data support. However, even Wampold and colleagues (Laska et al., 2014) concede that exposure is necessary for the treatment of some anxiety disorders.

What is the significance of studies that have found slightly greater efficacy for cognitive-behavioral treatments when outcome is assessed with disorder-specific symptom measures? Is this due to the cognitive-behavioral nature of these interventions, or to the fact that the interventions are problem-focused? Yulish et al. (2017) offer a meta-analysis comparing treatments of different theoretical orientations and examine whether the treatments were problem-focused or not. In some studies that found cognitive-behavioral therapy to be more effective the comparison treatments were designed not to be problem-focused. The comparison therapists were sometimes even dissuaded from a focus on symptoms and encouraged to simply be sympathetic, non-directive, and non-judgmental. One of the findings of the meta-analysis of Yulish et al. was that problem-focused treatments, regardless of theoretical orientation, were equivalently effective, and more effective than treatments that are not problem-focused. One could draw from this an obvious lesson: if treatment focuses on symptoms or specific problems, it will get better outcomes on symptom measures than a treatment that is not focused on symptoms. However, Yulish et al. see something more here, namely, that the focus on symptoms is part of a therapeutic frame in which patients' distress about their specific problems is taken seriously. This focus raises patients' expectations of benefit from the treatment, which enhances its efficacy.

Nevertheless, focus on specific symptoms is not necessarily the fundamental key to better therapy. As Wampold et al. (2017) note, "If reduction in symptoms of one specific disorder does not also increase quality of life, well-being, interpersonal relations, and ability to work and function in society, then such symptoms may well be surrogate measures" (i.e., they substitute for meaningful outcomes) (p. 22). Specific symptoms of a disorder may need to be addressed in some fashion to improve outcome, but not to the exclusion of broader aspects of the patient's life.

There are other ways to investigate the differential efficacy of treatments besides the direct comparison of two types of therapy. In component studies patients are randomly assigned to two conditions, one of which is missing a procedure present in the other. For example, a specific intervention such as psychoeducation is not included in one of two groups receiving cognitive-behavioral therapy, or transference interpretation is left out of a comparison group's psychodynamic treatment. The results of such studies generally show that the presence or absence of a specific technique makes no difference, again with the possible exception of a small difference with regard to targeted variables for some components (see Lambert, 2013; Wampold, 2001; Wampold & Imel, 2015).

Another avenue of investigation is to look at the factor of therapist adherence to and competence in delivery of specific treatments. If a particular treatment's techniques are what make the difference for outcome, then therapists who adhere more closely to the guidelines for delivering that treatment and deliver it more competently should have better outcomes. The evidence suggests that this is not the case (see Webb et al., 2010).

The search for specificity of therapeutic effects has also focused on the ways different treatments are thought to target different psychological processes or mechanisms underlying a disorder. That is, research has attempted to ascertain whether different treatments might have similar overall outcome effects but bring about these effects through different mechanisms of action. One well-designed study, the National Institutes of Mental Health Treatment of Depression Collaborative Research Program (Elkin et al., 1989), included efforts to assess the hypothesized mechanisms of action for the different treatments that were compared in the study. The cognitive therapy in the study was presumed to work by changing cognitive distortions, the interpersonal therapy by addressing interpersonal relations and role transitions, and the medication treatment (imipramine) by improving neuro-vegetative and somatic symptoms. None of these treatments showed this specificity of effect. The treatments brought about equivalent improvements in overall depressive symptomatology, but the different therapies did not have differential effects on the targeted underlying mechanisms (Imber et al., 1990). In his overview of this topic Kazdin (2007) finds little support for most hypothesized mechanisms of action in the different therapies.

Common Factors

If therapy is clearly efficacious, but there is relatively little difference in efficacy between treatments that employ different techniques, then what makes therapy efficacious? One explanation points to common factors, aspects of treatment that different therapies share. For example, every therapy involves a therapist and a patient engaged in a relationship of collaborative work intended to resolve the patient's problems. Therapists offer (at least implicitly through the practices of the therapy itself) some perspective on the problem and what would help to resolve it.

These and other general features have been studied extensively by psychotherapy researchers. One of the most frequently investigated common factors is the relationship between therapist and patient, often conceptualized in terms of the therapeutic alliance. Bordin (1979) conceptualized the alliance as consisting of agreement about the goals and tasks of therapy, as well as a bond between therapist and patient. Overall, measures of the alliance correlate well with outcome (Fluckiger et al., 2018; Martin et al., 2000). There are many subtleties to the research on the alliance, but they do not weaken the general finding of correlation between alliance and outcome. Some have questioned whether the alliance predicts outcome, hypothesizing that early symptomatic improvement may instead create a better alliance. Barber et al. (2000) found that symptom change does improve alliance, but that alliance is a significant predictor of further symptomatic improvement apart from any early decrease in symptoms.

Therapist empathy is clearly correlated with outcome. According to Wampold and Imel (2015), empathy "is more highly correlated with outcome than any other variable studied in psychotherapy" (p. 211; see also Elliott et al., 2018). While empathy is given theoretical importance in some therapies (client-centered therapy and self-psychology variants of psychoanalysis), it is not the preserve of any one type of therapy and is best understood as a common factor.

Several other common factors have been proposed. Grencavage and Norcross (1990) surveyed the literature and found the most frequently referenced common factors to include the alliance, the opportunity for catharsis, the acquisition and practice of new behaviors, clients' positive expectancies, beneficial therapist qualities, and the provision of a rationale for the patient's problems. Wampold and Imel (2015, pp. 256–259) summarize the research on the relative contributions to outcome of common factors and specific techniques. Their general conclusion is that several common factors have effects that are larger than the effects produced by specific ingredients of therapy, "a difference sometimes approaching an order of magnitude or more" (p. 256).

Psychotherapy as Healing Social Practice

The role of common factors in therapeutic efficacy has prompted some to abandon the conception of therapy as a set of technical interventions that target the underlying causes or maintaining features of disorders. Frank and Frank (1991) suggest that at the heart of the particular problems that people bring to therapy lies a sense of demoralization. Psychotherapy is primarily about re-moralizing people, helping them to feel less defeated and helpless in the face of their problems. Re-moralizing can be carried out through a variety of specific therapeutic methods. Whatever specific therapeutic techniques are being used there is always a patient engaged in a relationship with a socially recognized healer. The healer provides an explanation for the patient's problems and offers the patient some procedures that allow opportunities for experiences of success or mastery in the context of emotional arousal. Frank and Frank see these general aspects of therapy to be what is helpful, while no particular technical instantiation of them is necessary for therapy to work.

In an approach similar to and partly inspired by the Franks' model, Wampold (2001) and Wampold and Imel (2015) present a picture of therapy as a healing social practice. Their contextual model proposes three pathways through which therapy is helpful. First, if an initial bond is made (a sense of being able to engage with the therapist, and trust that the therapist can help), then a real relationship can develop. The latter includes a sense of the genuineness of both participants, the feeling that the patient can be open and honest with the therapist, and the sense that the therapist is empathic.

Second, therapy is efficacious through the expectation of benefit it creates. What matters here is patients' acceptance of both the therapist's explanations for their problems, and the reasonableness of the procedures to be engaged in. It is crucial that the patient have a sense that the therapist has something specific to offer that will make a difference. "One of the common factors is the systematic use of some set of specific ingredients, delivered in a cogent and convincing manner to the client and accepted by the client" (Wampold & Imel, 2015, p. 59).

Third, while it is necessary that the therapy have specific ingredients, the reason such specifics are helpful is not that they target the underlying psychological deficits of the patient. Rather, the specific procedures of the various therapies change *something* in a positive direction. What a therapy focuses on changing will vary widely (cognitive distortions, self-destructive behaviors, avoidance of particular types of interpersonal engagement or of certain emotions, wishes, fantasies, etc.). But change in one area tends to generalize to others. Overcoming avoidance of anxiety-provoking situations may improve self-esteem. Experiencing and owning hostile feelings and fantasies in therapy sessions can lead to greater capacity to be assertive outside therapy.

Two Readings of the Research: Atomistic and Holistic

So there are two fundamental approaches to the psychotherapy research, with correspondingly different conceptions of what therapy is. In one approach psychological problems are conceptualized as suitable for analysis into underlying factors that can be changed through targeted intervention. The other emphasizes the meaning of human experience in its social context, considering how trust, empathy, hope, and expectation are strengthened through specific interventions with cogent rationales.

How should we understand this fundamental difference? The conflict is rooted in contrasting conceptions of the nature of psychological problems, of psychotherapy, and of how the latter addresses the former. One approach seeks to identify specifiable psychological processes (for example, the conditioning of autonomic arousal in panic or cognitive distortions in depression) that can be changed through interventions that target them (interoceptive exposure or rational testing of automatic thoughts). The other approach claims that what is most fundamental to therapy are experiences of sense-making, expectations of help, and being empathically understood, phenomena that can be present in any therapy regardless of hypothesized underlying processes that are directly targeted. One approach views psychological problems in individualistic-atomistic terms as self-contained psychological processes within the individual that are targeted by the treatment. The other approach understands psychological phenomena in social-holistic terms as contextually shaped and socially or interpersonally addressed through empathic understanding and joint sense-making.

These fundamentally different approaches to psychological phenomena lead to a rather striking miscomprehension of one view by the other. What is important to note is that the miscomprehension tends to occur in only one direction. Frank and Frank's (1991) hermeneutic-rhetorical model of therapy and Wampold and Imel's (2015) contextual model were developed to respond to the standard individualistic-atomistic model that is the lingua franca of psychotherapy research. It is difficult to make sense of the social-holistic model when examined through the assumptions of the standard model. Those subscribing to the standard individualistic model can of course acknowledge that there are data to support the efficacy of common factors such as the alliance, even if they may dispute how important they are (Chambless & Crits-Christoph, 2006). But there is a tendency to characterize such factors in atomistic terms. That is, the alliance and other common factors are conceptualized as efficacious elements of treatment that happen to be present in many types of therapy and either correct some specific psychological deficit within the patient or support the delivery of other interventions that do. There are a number of misunderstandings generated by the effort to subsume the social-holistic approach within an individual-atomistic framework. The distinctive features of each approach can be clarified by examining some of these misunderstandings.

First Misunderstanding

The social-holistic perspective on therapy is mischaracterized as claiming that all one need do in therapy is utilize common factors, with no consideration of anything specific to patients or their particular problems. The argument is then made that this won't work, that we cannot dissolve all the specific interventions of different therapies into common factors such as an empathic positive alliance between therapist and patient. Recommendations for treatment can't simply be to have a good relationship with one's patient, and then do the same therapy with everyone, whether the person is suffering from schizophrenia, alcohol dependence, or social anxiety (see Hoffman & Barlow, 2014).

Response: Those who attribute a greater role to common than specific factors are not suggesting that one need never adapt a therapy to the particular problems of the patient. All therapies have to be adapted to the particulars of patients' problems, as well as to their broader personal characteristics, their intellectual abilities, to their financial resources, or levels of social support. But this is a requirement incumbent upon all types of therapy, not an argument for doing one type of therapy, or one specific set of therapeutic procedures, rather than another. Both psychodynamic therapy (e.g., Bateman & Fonagy, 2004; Clarkin, Yeomans & Kernberg, 1999; Kernberg et al., 1989) and cognitive-behavioral therapy (Linehan, 1993; Neacsiu & Linehan, 2014) were adapted for work with borderline personality disorder. But the changes to these therapies did not result in their becoming essentially the same treatment using the same techniques. After modification to address the particular difficulties associated with borderline disorder, they each remain clearly recognizable examples of distinct therapeutic orientations.

The emphasis on common factors in the social-holistic approach does not entail that there is no need to adapt treatments to the particulars of patient and problem. But neither does the modification of different therapies to address specific problems lead to all therapies looking alike. Common factors are operative across technique and problem. They do not subsume and dissolve all specifics into one common therapy for all disorders.

Second Misunderstanding

Social-holistic approaches to therapy are incorrectly seen as aiming at the same therapeutic goals as therapies that fit the individualistic-atomistic model. There is some evidence for advantages to cognitive-behavioral therapy in the treatment of depression and anxiety when outcome is assessed with disorder-specific measures. Since getting better outcomes of this sort is what we all want, it is incumbent upon all therapies to consist of specific interventions that achieve results like these.

Response: Specific interventions aim at specific targets. From a social-holistic perspective, the aims of therapy need not be so narrowly conceived. Why should symptom measures carry so much weight? The emphasis on concrete symptoms does not just make for more easily measurable outcome scores. This emphasis also implies that such symptoms are definitive of psychological distress. This view of psychological disorder entails assumptions about therapeutic aims, about what benefits are most valuable for their patients, where their good lies. Shedler (2010) has critiqued standard research for its narrow focus on symptoms as *the* measure of outcome. Why not consider outcome measures that examine other components of living a rich and satisfying life? He proposes that therapy be assessed for whether it promotes:

> Greater satisfaction in pursuing long-term goals, enjoyment of challenges and pleasure in accomplishments, ability to utilize talents and abilities, contentment in life's activities, empathy for others, interpersonal assertiveness and effectiveness, ability to hear and benefit from emotionally threatening information, and resolution of past painful experiences.
>
> (pp. 105–106)

Therapies may have aims that go beyond symptom reduction. Further, a focus on symptomatic change can even impede those broader aims. For example, Ogden and Gabbard (2010) argue that a focus on symptoms can lead to impasses in an analytic treatment that tries to help "the patient get to know and accept himself as the broadened and deepened subject he becomes in the course of the analysis" (p. 543).

Third Misunderstanding

The focus on common factors can be unfavorably compared to a focus on specific techniques by taking up questions of practical utility and "portability." Skills for monitoring and fostering the alliance or empathy are subtle, depend on personal characteristics of therapists, and are not easily taught. It's a far more manageable task to teach a therapist a protocol for psychoeducation, or for how to help patients assess the evidence regarding whether panic attacks are truly dangerous. Unlike understanding the subtleties of relationship, techniques can be more easily disseminated, bringing their benefits to more patients through the straightforward training of greater numbers of therapists (see Baker & McFall, 2014).

   Response: The misunderstanding here is a confusion of what's readily doable with what's worth doing. The fundamental values of efficacy and efficiency that are sought in some treatments are here applied to the dissemination of those treatments and the training of therapists. But if common factors make a significant contribution to outcome, why not do the work to train therapists to be attentive to their role in therapy? It's true that empathy and sensitivity to the state of the alliance build on personal qualities of therapists. Enhancing such skills involves personal development, not just the imparting of information about how to do specific techniques. A social-holistic view of therapy involves aims for patients that are broader than symptom reduction and aims for therapists that are broader than the mastery of techniques.

Fourth Misunderstanding

This miscomprehension is evident in several of the responses to an article summarizing common factors research in the December 2014 issue of the journal *Psychotherapy* (Laska et al., 2014). Crits-Christophe et al. (2014) propose testing the common factors perspective on therapy by turning it into a testable treatment. They argue that if such treatment passes the test of a randomized controlled trial it could turn out to be another empirically supported treatment. Asnaani and Foa (2014) also call for a head-to-head comparison of "an active, disorder specific treatment ... against a treatment that includes *only* common factors" (p. 488).

Response: These suggestions misunderstand the central idea of the social-holistic conception of therapy. This conception of therapy claims that the efficacy of any treatment offering any of a variety of means to change a variety of disorders is largely the result of common factors that will be present in any of those therapies (this is why such different treatments can have equivalent outcomes). Common factors are seen as underlying all of the specific interventions and their presumed specific modes of action on whatever is causing or maintaining the psychopathology. One cannot do a "disorder-specific treatment" that does not include common factors. Nor can one do a "common factors treatment" that includes no specific procedures. Even if common factors must take *some* specific form, the common factors can't be identified with a specific set of forms. There are no definitive scientific categories that can delimit these forms because of the fluidity of contexts that determine whether something said or done by a therapist is, for example, empathic or alliance-building. For one patient in one context a sarcastic comment on the therapist's part could be experienced as a humorous and gentle confrontation that strengthens the bond between them. For another (or the same patient on another occasion) a sarcastic comment could be experienced as demeaning and destructive to the therapy. It is unlikely that anyone will be able to come up with a set of therapeutic procedures that constitutes *the* method for strengthening the alliance. According to Constantino and Bernecker (2014), even some advocates for empirically supported treatments are beginning to recognize that the key to good therapy is not the strict application of specific interventions but adaptations that reinvent procedure in light of what is relevant to the clinical situation at hand.

Problems with an Atomistic Approach

What lies at the heart of the skepticism about developing specific treatments for specific problems? It is not simply the pragmatic difficulties in testing each of the myriad therapies for the continually multiplying number of psychiatric disorders. This pragmatic problem makes it appear as though the difficulty were the number of comparative studies that would need to be done (does technique T reduce symptom S in disorder D for patients with characteristics C1, C2, and C3, etc.?). But complexity of that sort is present in many sciences. More problematic is the fact that psychological factors lack stability and take on specific meaning only within specific contexts. Further, the range of relevant contexts is difficult to delimit conceptually or naturalistically. The meaning of any particular behavior or psychological phenomenon can only be ascertained holistically.[2] Understanding therapeutic change entails attention to the contextually determined meanings of what is changed, which do not sort neatly into stable categories.

By contrast, meteorological prediction is certainly complex, but at least there are some fundamental factors that have a consistent meaning with standard measures. Temperature, wind speed, barometric pressure, and humidity provide some consistent and measurable core factors in the efforts to model and predict the weather. In chemistry there is a periodic table of the elements. There is no psychological equivalent to the periodic table of the elements. Scientific psychology may have provided evidence for some fundamental components of psychological life, such as a list of basic emotions, or the significance of attachment needs, or consistent patterns of habituation to arousal. But how these show up in the therapist's office is so complexly interwoven with the meanings they have for patients, with how they fit into the broader contexts of their lives, that they don't provide a clear-cut scientific basis for how to intervene.[3] Further, the contexts that shape the meanings of particular behaviors also shift in ways that create new categories of meaning, changing the nature of the psychological problems that patients present.

For example, consider how a basic emotion like anger may appear as the partly genuine, partly performative righteous indignation of a politician, or as the unrestrained protective anger of a mother toward someone bullying her child. Or consider a controlled testiness in response to a perceived affront to the dignity of a patrician Anglican cleric, compared to the quick, "hot" aggressive move to put down a high school rival by a student athlete. It is the different meanings of these contextually embedded forms of anger that the psychotherapist needs to be sensitive to. The basic science provides little help, nor does it provide scientifically definable categories of anger that are of much use to the therapist. The part played by social identity, role, or class (patrician cleric, high school rivals) in giving shape to these different angers is further transformed when one looks at different cultures. Contrast these two cases: (1) the angry response to an affront to the dignity of an Anglican cleric supervising a youth group in working class London; and (2) the restrained fury ("Oh, God, here it is again!") of the African-American teacher who has been told by a white school administrator that he just assumed she'd develop activities for Black History Month. The therapist's job is not simply to identify another instance of a basic emotion—both of them know they are angry. The therapist's task is to explore with them difficult binds that arise with these complicated feelings. They may find themselves uncertain about what to do with the anger they continue to feel, with shame that they didn't address the offense more directly, with fear about the reaction to their anger—or all of the above at once. Exploring such a complicated situation can't be done without sensitivity to the broader social contexts of what it means for this upper class Englishman to be serving working class youth as an Anglican priest, or what it means for the teacher to hear the administrator frame Black History Month as the exclusive business of African Americans, that is, as having nothing to do with him.

It is not just social or political context that matters. Therapists are often attuned to the details of how patients' personal histories shape the significance of emotional experience and expression. The tendency of one patient's father to take a condescending tone with him, especially in front of his mother, gives a particular meaning to the rage that he feels (and suppresses) when slighted in mixed company. By contrast, the danger one woman felt of being icily cut off if she ever became angry with her mother gives a context for her obsessively trying to please others, and for feeling despair when her anger slips out. Again, it is these nuances that therapists attend to, and the science of basic emotions is little help in attending to them.

Further, there are intra-therapeutic contexts that shape the meaning of what a patient is saying or experiencing. How therapists listen, what therapists are capable of or interested in hearing, will shape what patients have to say and how they say it. This is obvious if one contrasts very different therapies. Patients in more structured therapies that are focused on skills for identifying and changing symptoms or problematic behaviors learn to talk about instances of success or failure in the development of such skills. Patients in psychodynamic therapy learn that attention to what is passing through their minds, or to how they are responding to their therapists, is central to what this therapy is about (even when they resist paying attention to these). But the contexts that influence what is said or done and what it means can be far more subtle. Donnell Stern (1997, 2010, 2015, 2019) has written extensively on how enactments in psychoanalytic therapy constrict what both patient and analyst are capable of bringing into the room. The enactments of analyst and patient create a context that locks in place certain meanings, affects, or ways of relating to one another and makes others impossible. Correlatively, moving out of such enactments opens up new possibilities. "It is the immediate human context between patient and analyst that determines what they can experience in one another's presence" (Stern, 2019, p. 10).

These multiple forms of context dependence do not mean that scientific research can tell us nothing about any specifics relevant to psychotherapy. There are mountains of papers presenting the results of such research. What I am disputing is that research provides evidence that therapeutic practice is simply an application of psychological science. As Woolfolk and Murphy (2004) put it,

> The claim that therapy is not a science should be sharply distinguished from the claim, which all parties may happily concede, that therapy may draw on empirical study and have measurable, scientifically evaluable effects. Those properties of therapy do not make it a science, though: professional sports share them.
>
> (p. 170)

For example, research may tell us something about what's going on when therapists are sensitively attending to their patients, without telling therapists how to do so. Schore (2012) has explored the relevance of research in attachment theory and the neurobiology of affect regulation to therapists' attunement to their patients. He writes of how

> the empathic clinician's psychobiologically attuned right brain tracks at a preconscious level, not only the arousal rhythms and flows of the patient's affective states but also her own somatic countertransferential, interoceptive, and bodily based affective responses to the patient's implicit facial, prosodic, and gestural communications.
>
> (p. 41)

It is important to note that Schore calls this a preconscious activity. At times he describes it as even further from consciousness, referring to the therapist's "unconscious right mind" (p. 41). The idea of turning this into a deliberate technique would miss the point. He concludes:

> Thus, at the most essential level, the intersubjective work of psychotherapy is not defined by what the therapist does for the patient, or says to the patient (left brain focus). Rather, the key mechanism is how to be with the patient, especially during affectively stressful moments (right brain focus).
>
> (p. 44)

Some psychotherapy researchers have suggested that this kind of attunement or responsiveness to patients provides the central benefit of therapy, and that this helps to explain the equivalent effectiveness of contrasting techniques (see Stiles, 2009; Stiles et al., 1998).

Can this kind of attunement become the basis for a specific intervention, a deliberately applied technique? This kind of sensitivity is partly a function of character, partly developed through a stance of listening that opens therapists to a range of experiences with patients that helps to refine their responsiveness. Knowing that right brain processes underlie this capacity doesn't teach therapists how to do it. In fact, to the extent that one tries to develop a means to "do empathy" one is in danger of slipping into left brain thinking in a way that obscures or even impedes the right brain processes of attunement that happen without being directly willed.[4]

There are things the therapist can do that make a difference to empathy. Careful examination of what is happening in therapy may point a therapist toward a new perspective that brings about a shift in how the therapist feels toward the patient. Consider a therapist musing with one of her colleagues about something that feels "off" in her therapy with a patient:

> I've been annoyed the last couple of sessions. He seems to be presenting his distress as that of a helpless victim, and I'm feeling correspondingly critical—I want him to stop it ... But now I'm remembering that two sessions ago I felt some misgivings about how I responded to one of his disappointments—I think I was dismissive. Has he upped the ante of distress in response to that? Maybe I've been walling myself off from him in some way.

Now the therapist is feeling more curious and interested than annoyed. Her musings are not abstractly directed by principles, but guided by a felt sense (Gendlin, 1996) about the therapy. This reflection on what has been happening in the therapy helps to shift the therapist's perspective. The therapist then finds herself feeling differently. She does not generate the feeling directly. Her reflection enables her to step back from her emotional reaction to her patient, creating a space in which other feelings could arise. In McGilchrist's (2009) language, one could say that the therapist's attempt to examine what was amiss was an instance of the left brain appropriately serving the right, without usurping the right brain processes that remain outside direct control and that are more fundamental.[5]

When I speak of the meaning of psychological phenomena as dependent on context, and that the contexts that lend meaning are themselves multiple and shifting, I don't mean to suggest that there are no points of anchorage here. If there were no limits to the possible contexts that could illuminate what a patient is saying or doing, and if those contexts were constantly changing, patient and therapist would be lost in a swirling fog of meanings that were ultimately meaningless. In the immediacy of doing therapy, the therapist has to make choices about what to do, even if the decision is for the moment to do or say nothing. And how would the therapist make a choice without some sense that for this patient, at this moment, this context (and not that one) is the relevant one. There are moment-to-moment contexts that matter here, as well as the contexts of early versus late in treatment, the context of diagnosis, the context of the state of the alliance, the context of the patient's cultural background, the context of the therapist's approach to therapy, etc. The therapist's task here is to make a call as to which is the relevant context for this moment in therapy. Actually, the phrase "to make a call" makes this sound like a calculated choice. More often therapists find themselves responding to their patients and have a sense after the fact that a response was helpful or not. Certainly, the task is not simply to apply well-established psychological facts to a particular situation because the latter seems to fit a general category.

Therapists will differ on how they read contexts. Their reading of what is going on at a given moment in therapy, and of what is needed from them (just listen, educate, interpret, etc.) will be shaped by their psychological or therapeutic theories, of course. But it will also be shaped by subtleties of the moment that no theory or set of psychological facts can encompass. Psychoeducation is a component of many shorter term therapies, and the content is offered as scientific information that will be useful to the patient. And sometimes it is. But the therapist has to be paying attention to the patient to see how it is being received. If while explaining the fight-or-flight response to a patient with panic attacks there is a sneer on the patient's face (or a hostile stare and clenched fists, or the patient begins to cry) the truth of the facts about fight and flight are irrelevant. Something more than information about panic is called for here.[6]

Not all contexts are so readily apparent. Consider this clinical situation. A therapist has been working with a patient who has been trying to understand the way he constantly second guesses himself, especially when a decision he has made could be interpreted by himself or others as self-serving. He begins a session talking of a situation like many that have been discussed before, where he chose to stand his ground for something he thought was fair both to himself and to another party. He describes how soon after this decision was made he began to feel anxious and criticize himself for what he had done, a self-critique that was familiar from prior sessions. But the therapist did not step forward to explore what had happened the way that she had with previous incidents like this. She just listened. And before long the patient remarked on how his second guessing was short-lived this time. He let it go relatively quickly. He then went on to talk of how his wife has recently com-mended him for being more direct with her, straightforwardly asking her for what he wants, even though she doesn't always like what she hears.

Why did the therapist do something different this time? It is not clear that it would have been wrong to respond the way she had in previous sessions, asking for the details of what happened, exploring the various features of his self-critique. Did she sense something in the patient, a less tense, easier way of telling the story that indicated to her she should simply let him go on, that he didn't need her assistance in trying to understand it? Giving him room to tell the story at his own pace seemed to be the right thing to do. There was some reading of context, perhaps of his emotional tone, that led her to step back. In retrospect she not only noticed she did something different, but that it seemed right, and even suggested to her that she could do more of this in future sessions. She wondered if she had recently been working too hard to help him not to be so hard on himself. Reading the relevant context in this case is not something one can predict. She did not directly generate it from a theory. It just felt right. Even if one of the operative contexts that made it feel right was a theory that has influenced her, something in the moment called up its relevance. She needed to not just have a theory, but to read the moment in such a way as to bring the right aspect of the theory to bear (preconsciously, as Schore notes). One can do this well or poorly; there is a skill here that can be developed. But it is like the skill of reading literature perceptively or of jazz improvisation—it is not a set of techniques. One might also compare this to Aristotelian ideas about practical wisdom (see Smith, K. R., 2009). And if the literature on the general equivalence of therapies is correct, very different therapies, based on different theories, utilizing different techniques, can all be the basis for skilled therapeutic reading of the relevant context.

Treatment Effects and Ethical Aspirations

The shifting and multi-layered contexts that shape psychological phenomena are one reason to challenge the picture of therapy as the application of effec-tive techniques to symptom-defined disorders. Reading those contexts skill-fully can lead therapists to useful but unpredictable responses to ongoing and changing events in session. But there is another reason for skepticism about the idea that therapy is a targeted intervention based on psychological sci-ence. What therapists do in therapy is not simply employ effective procedures that act upon patients. Therapy also includes an appeal to patients to take on particular ways of viewing themselves and their problems. Something is held out to the patient as a better way to think about their difficulties, some-times re-defining them or suggesting a different direction in which to look for improvement.

Insofar as therapy is offering patients a different understanding of what is amiss, a different idea about how to make things better, even a different idea about *what* would be better, it is doing more than acting upon them in such a way as to change them. It is suggesting to patients a different way of looking at themselves that includes a different perspective on where their well-being lies. Therapy does not bring about change just through influences that operate upon people, but through appealing to aspirations for a better life.

This may seem obvious, but it is often overlooked in the search for explanations of psychological problems and how to treat them. The standard investigation of therapeutic efficacy (what works for which problems, for which patients, and how and why) will conceive of the human aspiration for something better as a motivational factor in the patient that operates as another efficient cause. When conceptualized as another causal factor, its evaluative import is stripped away. "The good aimed at" is translated into a psychological event or factor of "aiming at the good" that can be used as a means to some other end.[7] It no longer matters whether the good is good, or that it is good. All that matters is whether the patient believes it is good and that this state of believing is causally effective in bringing about a psychological change such as a decrease in symptoms. Approached in this way, the therapist is locked out of either taking up the patient's notion of the good for consideration with the patient, or stepping aside to allow the patient's pursuit of the good to carry them forward (which is a sort of endorsement of it). Instead, the therapist can only either ignore it or manipulate the patient's belief in it as a potentially efficacious factor.

As Taylor (2007b) puts it, in this understanding of therapy, people "are just to be dealt with, manipulated into health" (p. 620). Instead of seeing the problems that people bring to therapy as part of an effort to find a good life, an effort that has gone awry, they are viewed as signs of a condition that needs to be treated, managed, or therapeutically altered. On this view, the therapist is not a fellow traveler who is also a seeker of the good life, and understands patients' troubles in that context. Instead, the therapist is an expert who knows how to alter those conditions in patients that have generated these symptoms or disorders. Repair of these limiting conditions will enable patients to go on to pursue whatever forms of life appeal to them. From this perspective, therapy ought not to take up any questions, even indirectly, about what constitutes human well-being. But this hands-off stance toward questions of human flourishing can be part of an implicit, constricted picture of well-being as the absence of symptoms or disorder: there is nothing more to aspire to. What brought the patient into therapy (anxiety, depression, or other symptoms) has nothing to do with any aspirations beyond being free of these symptoms.

Taylor's (2007b) discussion of "the therapeutic" (building on Rieff, 1966) may draw too stark a contrast between therapy and ethical or spiritual aspirations to a good life. He suggests that many therapists would respond to a patient who was "a highly successful professional, with a high income, feeling an uneasy sense that something crucial was missing in his life" (p. 622) by assuming that the only task at hand was simply to relieve the unease. On the contrary, there are a number of therapeutic theorists who would see psychopathology not just in this patient's anxiety, but in his living a high-functioning but constricted and dispirited life. This is the significance of Bollas's (1987) writing on normotic illness, Fromm's (1976) on the marketing personality, and Fink's (2007) on the non-normalizing aims of psychoanalysis. Nevertheless, it is true that therapists rarely allow themselves to use the language of ethics in a full sense. They are often more comfortable with the language of repair (whether this is couched as the repair of a disorder, or the repair of the deforming experiences of childhood in the context of family dynamics), than the language of ethical aspirations for a good life.[8]

There is a risk that arises with the conception of therapy as the utilization by the therapist of the results of research into what makes therapy efficacious. The risk is that therapists do not stand beside their patients in their search for a better life, but only act upon them in the effort to remove psychological obstacles in their paths. I am not suggesting that the latter is always inappropriate. But it does not encompass the ways in which therapy also offers patients its own conceptions of flourishing.

Further, approaching psychotherapy as an intervention intended to bring about symptomatic improvement can sideline aspects of ethics that can't be conceptualized in terms of effective means to an end. Consider positive psychology's gratitude exercises (Seligman, 2011; Seligman et al., 2005), which have been shown to improve mood (at least in the short term). I have no doubt that people can benefit significantly from reminding themselves of what they have to be grateful for. But the idea of making an act of gratitude a technique for boosting one's mood risks undermining the gratitude. Imagine someone saying, "I'm glad to thank you for what you've done for me, because I understand that thanking you will make me feel happy." Aside from the effect on the person to whom this is said, there is a way in which this hollows out the gratitude. If I am truly grateful to someone this includes a sense that it is right to be grateful, a perception that this person has been good to me, that I ought not to take that for granted, and perhaps that I owe the person some sign of my gratitude. To shift from a focus upon my own agendas toward a stance of gratitude is to re-orient my perspective on what matters. What is good about gratitude in this sense is missing when it is turned into a technique for feeling happy. This is not to suggest that there is something wrong with feeling better because one has done the right thing. But if all I know about gratitude is that it feels good, if I don't know that it is the right response to having been given something beyond what I can claim as owed to me, then whatever I'm doing when I say that I am grateful, I'm not grateful.

Summary

I have presented the results of a number of psychotherapy research studies and considered various arguments and counterarguments regarding their significance. The conclusions can be summarized as follows.

The research comparing different types of treatments and techniques shows little evidence of difference in efficacy between them (with perhaps a few exceptions). Some believe that continued search for effective techniques is still worth pursuing, perhaps supplementing techniques with attention to useful common factors. Others call for a fundamental re-conceptualization of what therapy is. This revised view of therapy sees it not as an instrumental means to bring about a specific end, but as engaging people in practices that enact new meanings through affectively charged experiences. These affectively enacted new meanings often include changes in patients' perspectives on what matters, on what's worthwhile for living a full and flourishing life. Further, this fundamental therapeutic process is not tied to a particular therapy but can be carried out in a variety of treatments with divergent techniques and theoretical foundations.

Finally, I argued that there are significant limitations to the conception of therapy as a set of efficacious techniques. The effort to specify particular symptoms and disorders treated by an empirically supported package of specific interventions relies on an atomistic picture of psychological phenomena. I proposed that psychological phenomena are better approached holistically, as interdependent with a variety of contexts (the context of personal history; of current interpersonal setting; of social, historical, and cultural environment, etc.). Running through these contexts are ideas regarding what matters most for living well, ideas that orient both patients and therapists. A conception of therapy as a technical intervention to achieve a circumscribed goal can lead to the development of powerful techniques. But it can also obscure the ethical component of therapy, or promote one ethical aim (that of effective self-control) over others, without acknowledging that it is doing so.

I want to emphasize one final point that is central to the themes of the preceding two chapters. If the different types of therapy (psychodynamic, cognitive-behavioral, humanistic, etc.) and the different techniques nested within them are generally equivalent in efficacy, why do therapists remain wedded to their respective approaches? What I tried to show in Chapters 3 and 4 is that adherence to favored therapeutic orientations is influenced by the appeal of the particular picture of flourishing, of how to live life well and fully, that is part of a therapy's ethos. The role that ideas of well-being play in the attachment to particular therapeutic approaches has consequences for how to read the literature on efficacy. The standard question about whether a therapy works needs to be supplemented by examining what picture of flourishing it serves. However, this not only complicates the project to develop treatments with empirically supported techniques (the "psychological treatments" described by Barlow, 2004), but leaves important questions unanswered by the social-holistic understanding of therapy as well.

Which Therapy? A Dilemma for the Social-Holistic Approach

Compared to the individualistic-atomistic approach, the social-holistic conception of therapy can more easily make room for the evaluative dimension of human experience. Examining psychological problems in social context inevitably involves consideration of socially valued goods. But this approach is not without its own problems. Frank and Frank (1991) note that while every therapy needs to have some "rationale, conceptual scheme, or myth that provides a plausible explanation for the patient's symptoms and prescribes a ritual or procedure for resolving them" (p. 42), there is no indication or evidence to suggest that this rationale must be empirically founded. Wampold (2001) addresses the concern that the finding of uniform efficacy across very different types of therapy could be taken as support for religious or occult rationales for psychotherapy. He claims that we need not worry about this because "psychologists are bound by a profession imbedded in the science of psychology" (p. 223). While this is perhaps the politically correct thing to say to his fellow researchers, it doesn't change the fact that the results of research give no grounds for sticking to scientifically supported rationales for therapy. This is why Frank and Frank state that a myth will do.

Wampold acknowledges this in other work (Benish, Quintana, & Wampold, 2011; Wampold, 2007) in which he doesn't raise concerns about the non-scientific basis for myths that are consonant with the patient's worldview or culture. The question still remains whether therapists wouldn't have to have at least a partial endorsement of the myth themselves. Few therapists (I hope) would join with someone's racist explanations for despair and hopelessness ("My life's a mess because blacks and immigrants have all the advantages") in order to deepen a patient's self-understanding or to further acceptance of a particular therapeutic approach. There are atheists and scientifically minded therapists who would feel dishonest or at least disingenuous talking with patients in religious terms about their problems. To speak with the patient in terms of a myth that is believable to the patient but that the therapist is skeptical about or appalled by--would this not undermine the therapist's capacity to engender the positive expectations of improvement that boost therapeutic success?

Further, if therapists were able to positively influence patients by going along with a mythological frame that the therapist didn't believe in, would this make therapy a "sales job" or con game? Would the idea implicitly be that one should talk to patients in terms they already subscribe to, whether the therapist believes them or not, in order to get patients to buy in to the therapy? Granted that therapists need to be willing to look at the patient's dilemmas through a worldview that is not the therapist's own, are there no limits to this? Is it ever legitimate for the therapist to move in a different direction, where the patient's myths, values, or worldview are subject to re-examination? If so, how? How direct a challenge can this be? Can therapy ever legitimately be an ethical debate or "instruction," or would this not be counter to a fundamental therapeutic ethic, counter to most therapists' under-standing of what therapy is and does? If so, what does this ethic tell us about therapy?

Aside from the difficulties that arise when there is a conflict between therapist and patient "myths," therapists have the problem of deciding about their own therapeutic theory. Eysenck (1993) complains that if all types of therapy were indeed uniformly efficacious (and it is clear that he does not believe that they are) then it would surely spell "the definite rebuttal to all the theories psychotherapists have fought so earnestly to elaborate and establish" (p. 12). There would be no reason to do one type of therapy rather than another. In a review of the first edition of Wampold's *The Great Psychotherapy Debate*, Horvath et al. (2002) acknowledge that Wampold is not suggesting that thera-pists can utilize any theory or myth they wish, no matter how outlandish. Nevertheless, they go on to raise a basic issue. "Without making clear what makes a theory plausible and a 'therapeutic ritual' legitimate, we are faced with the question: On what basis should the therapist commit her or his alle-giance?" (p. 111).

So there are divergent opinions on this issue, with Frank and Frank being more comfortable with empirically unsupported myths as the rationale pro-vided for a therapy, others wanting a more solid scientific grounding for the reason to do one therapy rather than another.

According to the social-holistic understanding, a workable therapy needs a plausible, convincing rationale with accompanying believable therapeutic procedures. The rationales and procedures have to be plausible to therapists as well as patients. If therapists don't believe in it they are less likely to be able to foster believability in patients (this is one of the problems with compar-ing bona fide treatments to those that are not). Many therapists are inclined toward scientific foundations for the believable—so given who therapists are, they will seek scientific justifications for the therapy they do. But this is an inclination of therapists that is not itself scientifically justified. Further, what the science seems to justify at one time can change and then influence believability in ways that change a treatment's efficacy. For example, Johnsen and Friborg (2015) have found that over time cognitive-behavioral therapy has become less efficacious for the treatment of depression. They hypothesize that part of this decline is due to messaging about cognitive-behavioral therapy's effectiveness. That is, touting cognitive-behavioral therapy as the scientifically proven new therapy made it initially more convincing and hence more effective. Over time the luster of being "the newest and best" wore off and it became less impressive to people and therefore less effective. They hypothesize that their own paper showing its decline in effectiveness may damage the reputation of cognitive-behavioral therapy and further decrease its effectiveness.[9]

What do we say then in response to the question Horvath et al. (2002) posed for Wampold: On what basis should therapists commit their allegiance to a particular type of therapy? It would seem that there is nothing wrong with answering: It doesn't matter what therapists commit their allegiance to, as long as therapist and patient both find the therapy believable, on any basis whatsoever.

But this seems to miss something important about psychotherapy, and about belief. When therapists decide that psychodynamic ways of thinking about people make more (or less) sense than cognitive-behavioral or humanistic ones, it cannot appear completely arbitrary to them. If it were arbitrary, how could they believe in it? Nor is this an accurate picture of how therapists develop particular therapeutic allegiances. Therapists are drawn to a particular therapy because it seems right, because it seems to make more sense of who people are, or addresses more important aspects of who people are, or because of their own positive experiences with it as patient or therapist. What the foregoing research suggests is that the data regarding therapeutic efficacy provide little support for a therapist's endorsement of a particular approach. If research were the only legitimate support for allegiance, then Horvath et al. (2002) would be right to question whether allegiance to a particular orientation can have a rational basis.

If it is suggested that the therapist should not have allegiance to a particular school of therapy but only to treatments or techniques that work, regardless of school, this too is a particular allegiance. It is allegiance to an ethic that claims that effectiveness at symptom reduction is all that really matters in helping patients to improve their lives. The prior two chapters examined how therapies differ regarding fundamental conceptions of human life, of how life can go wrong for us, what we can aspire to, what shape given to a life makes it a good one, etc. Even those treatments that claim to aim only at symptomatic change include more sweeping ethical aspirations. The hope of many psychological scientists has been to develop a conception of psychopathology and health that prescinds from commitments to any particular ethic. I am proposing that there are no psychological facts relevant to psychotherapy that are totally divorced from ethics.

I hope to have shown by this point that the therapies inevitably engage ethics, that is, they include at least implicit proposals regarding what makes for a full and flourishing life. But this raises a number of questions. How can therapies promote particular ideas about living well when therapists are usually determined to respect patients' own choices about how to live their lives? Further, are there any central themes that recur in therapeutic visions of well-being or is each therapy promoting something unique? Where do therapeutic views of flourishing come from? Are they invented with the therapy, or do they have socio-historical roots that help to explain their salience and appeal? Finally, is there any recourse when ideas about a good life lead in different directions? Is reasoned ethical debate possible? I take up these questions in *Therapeutic Ethics in Context and in Dialogue*.

Notes

1 For an overview of the replication crisis in psychology, see Wiggins and Chrisopherson (2019).
2 See Dreyfus and Taylor (2015) for a discussion of the holistic nature of human meanings.
3 See Westen et al. (2004) on the "non-circumscribed" nature of most psychological problems.
4 See Aron's (2012) discussion of a therapist's efforts to *try* to be empathic precisely because she did not feel empathy but was horrified that her patient said he enjoyed the prospect of war following the 9/11 attacks.
5 For more in-depth discussion and examples of navigating emotional impasses between therapist and patient, see Safran and Muran (2000).
6 For a more detailed example of the necessity of modifying a cognitive-behavioral protocol, see Don et al. (2019).
7 See Brinkmann's (2011) critique of this way of psychologizing ethics.
8 I take up this reticence in *Therapeutic Ethics in Context and in Dialogue*, examining how ethics is present in therapy despite the reluctance to directly promote ideas about a good life.
9 This might be seen as a small-scale version of what Hacking (1995) refers to as "looping effects" in the social sciences, where people's knowledge of psychological facts changes those facts.

6 Conclusion
What Works? What Matters?

This study began with a few key ideas of Charles Taylor's philosophical anthropology. Persons are agents who are inevitably engaged in ethics. That is, they have ideas, implicit and explicit, about what is important in life, what makes a life worthwhile, what it is to live well. Further, where one stands on these questions about what matters partly constitutes the particular person one is. An ethical stance may not be fully articulated, or consistent, but the total absence of orientation to some good would represent a truncated mode of human existence. To see no good anywhere, to act without any conception of something worth aiming for, is hard to even imagine—under those conditions, why do anything at all? Our fellow animals show in their actions what matters to them. We are no different on that score.

Where we are distinct is in our ability to articulate our sense about what is worth pursuing in life, which also makes it possible to give shape to new conceptions of the good. These articulations happen in language. "Language" is understood broadly to include not just declarative statements and formal theories, but also social practices such as therapy and cultural expressions such as poetry, narrative, art, and symbols. Bringing our sense of the good to language in these ways is generative; it allows that sense to take on specific forms, to be revised and debated. It even makes it possible to question whether the whole process of trying to discover and articulate the good makes sense or is bound to lead to dead ends. It is an ethical investigation to inquire whether ethical investigation is worth the effort.

I have been exploring the implications of this view of persons for how we think about psychotherapy. In what way do fundamental concerns about what it means to live well enter into both the difficulties that people bring to therapy, and the therapy that aims to help them? Many have argued for a conception of psychotherapy as an intervention derived from psychological science that is used as a means to treat well-defined disorders or to change specific patterns of behavior and experience. As such, therapy would be no more of an ethical enterprise than orthopedic medicine or physical therapy. Psychotherapy would be seen as simply seeking to restore psychological health by treating mental disorders. I challenged this view in the third chapter, arguing that psychological problems are often intertwined with broader questions about what is important to a life well-lived. I also pointed to specific ethical ideals present even in therapies that are intended to be scientifically based treatments for circumscribed problems. Exposure-based behavioral therapy and cognitive therapy uphold the value of a scientific attitude that examines difficulties in living as analyzable into well-defined sub-problems with distinct causes, the mastery of which requires courage and enhances autonomy, self-efficacy, and independent thinking in the pursuit of one's freely chosen aims. These therapies are solidly rooted in a particular conception of what is essential to living well.

This is not a universally endorsed conception of human flourishing. Psychoanalysis was shown to promote a different ethic, where autonomy, for example, takes a different form or is sidelined altogether. Further, psychoanalysis does not present a united ethical stance, for different schools within it were shown to promote different ideas about flourishing.

The inevitable entanglement of therapeutic work with ethical aims has implications not just for how we understand what therapy is, but for how we assess its worth. The model of therapy as technical intervention for scientifically defined problems leads to an assessment of its efficacy in these terms, an assessment that forms the basis for designating some treatments as evidence-based. Research indicates that differential efficacy of treatments does not map onto different therapeutic orientations. Humanistic, cognitive-behavioral, psychodynamic, and other sorts of treatments are generally equivalently efficacious when assessed by standard means. This makes it all the more relevant to differentiate the therapies not on the basis of their success at symptom reduction but in terms of their different visions of what is most important in the effort to live a full and flourishing life.

Many people, both therapists and those seeking therapeutic help, have a basic sense that different schools of therapy offer different perspectives on human flourishing. But these differences are rarely part of formal discussions in the field regarding the merits of the psychotherapies. It is as though conceptions of human well-being were seen as outside the possibility for reasoned consideration if they can't be resolved through data regarding efficacy. However, the focus on empirical evidence for "what works" results in the elevation of one ethical value (efficacy at achieving delimited practical aims) over all others, without acknowledging that it is an ethic. Questions about whether a therapeutic goal is worth pursuing, or the best one to pursue, are often assumed to be already answered ("After all, no one wants to be depressed!"). Questions about the relative merits of broader ideas about human flourishing are seen as a matter of personal or cultural preference.

The idea seems to be that some people may like humanistic self-reflection or behavioral self-engineering, but there's no rational basis for choosing between them.

Even if this were true[1] it would still leave a major problem about psychotherapy unresolved. If we can't promote one therapy over another on the basis of its scientifically established greater efficacy at symptom change, and we can't give any reason to prefer one therapy's views of human well-being over another's, is choice of therapy just a coin toss (or a spin of the roulette wheel, since there are so many therapies)? I don't believe we should give up on the possibility of reasoned ethical discussion. The field could work harder to develop a discourse of ethical discernment and dialogue. Such discourse will not look like that of psychotherapy research, with relatively clear-cut measures of presumably ethically neutral objective criteria. The nature of ethics is such that it is essentially *not* neutral. Ethics makes claims that one mode of living is better than another. Ethical debate looks more like aesthetic or political debate than scientific dispute. Objective measures may play an important supportive or critical role but they won't help us to address core ethical differences.

Conversation between those holding contrasting visions of flourishing requires a willingness to explore more deeply others' contrasting views. This is not an easy task, not just because the issues are not resolvable with objective data, but because in truly engaging with another's ethic there is the possibility that one's own will be changed. And since personal identity is partly a function of ethics (who people are is partly a function of what they care most deeply about), such openness also entails the possibility of an identity cost. However, there is also the possibility of an identity gain as the encounter with the other broadens one's ethical perspective.

In order to be productive, conversation between different ethical views requires some effort to understand the contexts that lend plausibility to the other's ethical vision. These contexts are often particular social, cultural, and historical locations. Beyond this initial work of trying to understand the contexts for one another's perspectives lies the further task of speaking for one's own ethic while respectfully engaging with the other's take on what is most important for living a fulfilling life. I turn to these tasks in *Therapeutic Ethics in Context and in Dialogue*.

Note

1 In *Therapeutic Ethics in Context and in Dialogue* I argue that it is not.

References

American Psychological Association Division 12 Task Force. (1995). Training in dissemination of empirically validated psychological treatments: Report and recommendations. *The Clinical Psychologist, 48*, 3–23.

American Psychological Association. (2017). Ethical principles of psychologists and code of conduct. Retrieved December 27, 2019 from https://www.apa.org/ethics/code/.

Aristotle. (trans., 1984). Nichomachean ethics. In: J. Barnes (Ed.), *The Complete Works of Aristotle* (Vol. 2, pp. 1729–1867). Princeton, NJ: Princeton University Press.

Aron, L. (2012). Analytic impasse and the third: Clinical implications of intersubjectivity theory. In: L. Aron, & A. Harris (Eds.), *Relational Psychoanalysis* (Vol. 5, pp. 205–239). New York, NY: Routledge.

Aron, L., & Starr, K. (2013). *A Psychotherapy for the People: Toward a Progressive Psychoanalysis*. New York, NY: Routledge.

Asnaani, A., & Foa, E. B. (2014). Expanding the lens of evidence-based practice in psychotherapy to include a common factors perspective: Comment on Laska, Gurman, & Wampold. *Psychotherapy, 51*, 487–490. doi:10.1037/a0036891.

Atwood, G. E., & Stolorow, R. D. (1993). *Faces in a Cloud: Intersubjectivity in Personality Theory*. Northvale, NJ: Jason Aronson.

Baardseth, T. P., Goldberg, S. B., Pace, B. T., Wislocki, A. P., Frost, N. D., Siddiqui, J. R., Kivlighan, D. M., Laska, K. M., Del Re, A. C., Minami, T., & Wampold, B. E. (2013). Cognitive-behavioral therapy versus other therapies: Redux. *Clinical Psychology Review, 33*(3), 395–405. doi:10.1016/j.cpr.2013.01.004.

Baker, T. B., & McFall, R. M. (2014). The promise of science-based training and applicationin psychological clinical science. *Psychotherapy, 51*(4), 482–486. doi:10.1037/a0036563.

Barber, J. P., Connolly, M. B., Crits-Christoph, P., Gladis, L., & Siqueland, L. (2000). Alliancepredicts patients' outcome beyond in treatment change in symptoms. *Journal of Consulting and Clinical Psychology, 68*(6), 1027–1032. doi:10.1037/0022-006x.68.6.1027.

Barlow, D. H. (2002). *Anxiety and Its Disorders: The Nature and Treatment of Anxiety and Panic* (3rd ed.). New York, NY: Guilford Press.

Barlow, D. H. (2004). Psychological treatments. *American Psychologist*, *59*(9), 869–878. doi:10.1037/0003-66X.59.9.869.

Barlow, D. H. (Ed.) (2014). *Clinical Handbook of Psychological Disorders: A Step-By-Step Treatment Manual* (5th ed.). New York, NY: Guilford Press.

Barlow, D. H., & Craske, M. G. (2007). *Mastery of Your Anxiety and Panic* (4th ed.). New York, NY: Oxford University Press.

Bateman, A., & Fonagy, P. (2004). *Psychotherapy for Borderline Personality Disorder: Mentalization-Based Treatment*. New York, NY: Oxford University Press.

Beck, A. T., Rush, A. J., Shaw, B. F., & Emery, G. (1979). *Cognitive Therapy of Depression*. New York, NY: Guilford Press.

Benish, S. G., Imel, Z. E., & Wampold, B. E. (2008). The relative efficacy of bona fide pychotherapies for treating post-traumatic stress disorder: A meta-analysis of direct comparisons. *Clinical Psychology Review*, *28*(5), 746–748. doi:10.1016/j.cpr.2007.10.005.

Benish, S. G., Quintana, S., & Wampold, B. E. (2011). Culturally adapted psychotherapy and the legitimacy of myth: A direct-comparison analysis. *Journal of Counseling Psychology*, *58*(3), 279–289. doi:10:1037/a0023626.

Blatt, S. J. (2004). *Experiences of Depression: Theoretical, Clinical and Research Perspectives*. Washington, DC: American Psychological Association.

Bollas, C. (1987). *The Shadow of the Object: Psychoanalysis of the Unthought Known*. New York, NY: Columbia University Press.

Bordin, E. S. (1979). The generalizability of the psychoanalytic concept of the working alliance. *Psychotherapy: Theory, Research and Practice*, *16*(3), 252–260. doi:10.1037/h0085885.

Breuer, J., & Freud, S. (1955). On the psychical mechanism of hysterical phenomena: Preliminary communication. In: J. Strachey (Ed. & Trans.), *The Standard Edition of the Complete Psychological Works of Sigmund Freud* (Vol. 2, pp. 3–17). London: Hogarth Press. (Work originally published 1893).

Brinkmann, S. (2011). *Psychology as a Moral Science: Perspectives on Normativity*. New York, NY: Springer.

Chambless, D. L., & Crits-Christoph, P. (2006). The treatment method. In: J. C. Norcross, L. E. Beutler, & R. F. Levant (Eds.), *Evidence-Based Practices in Mental Health: Debate and Dialogue on Fundamental Questions* (pp. 191–200). Washington, DC: American Psychological Association.

Chambless, D. L., & Hollon, S. D. (1998). Defining empirically supported therapies. *Journal of Clinical and Consulting Psychology*, *66*(1), 7–18. doi:10.1037/0022-006X.66.1.7.

Clarkin, J. F., Yeomans, F. E., & Kernberg, O. F. (1999). *Psychotherapy for Borderline Personality*. New York, NY: John Wiley & Sons.

Constantino, M. J., & Bernecker, S. L. (2014). Bridging the common factors and empirically supported treatment camps: Comment on Laska, Gurman, and Wampold. *Psychotherapy*, *51*, 505–509. doi:10.1037/a0036604.

Crits-Christoph, P., Chambless, D. L., & Markell, H. M. (2014). Moving evidence-based practice forward successfully: Commentary on Laska, Gurman, and Wampold. *Psychotherapy*, *51*, 491–495. doi:10.1037/a0036508.

Cuijpers, P., Smit, F., Bohlmeijer, E., Hollon, S. D., & Andersson, G. (2010). Efficacy of cognitive-behavioral therapy and other psychological treatments for adult depression: Meta-analytic study of publication bias. *The British Journal of Psychiatry, 196*(3), 173–178. doi:10.1192/bjp.bp.109.066001.

Cushman, P. (1995). *Constructing the Self, Constructing America: A Cultural History of Psychotherapy.* Reading, MA: Addison-Wesley.

Cushman, P. (2019). *Travels with the Self: Interpreting Psychology as Cultural History.* New York, NY: Routledge.

de Waal, F. (2006). Morally evolved: Primate social instincts, human morality, and the rise and fall of "veneer theory". In: S. Macedo, & J. Ober (Eds.), *Primates and Philosophers: How Morality Evolved* (pp. 1–80). Princeton, NJ: Princeton University Press.

Dimen, M., & Goldner, V. (2005). Gender and sexuality. In: E. S. Person, A. M. Cooper, & G. O. Gabbard (Eds.), *Textbook of Psychoanalysis* (pp. 93–114). Washington, DC: American Psychiatric Publishing.

Don, F. J., Driessen, E., Molenaar, P. J., Spijker, J., & Dekker, J. J. M. (2019). Early interventions in cognitive behavioral therapy for depression: A study contrasting a low-adherent and a highly adherent case. *Psychotherapy, 56*(1), 48–54. doi:10.1037/pst0000219.

Dreyfus, H., & Taylor, C. (2015). *Retrieving Realism.* Cambridge, MA: Harvard University Press.

Elkin, I., Shea, T., Watkins, J. T., Imber, S. D., Sotsky, S. M., Collins, J. F., Glass, D. R., Pilkonis, P. A., Leber, W. R., & Parloff, M. B. (1989). National Institute of Mental Health treatment of Depression Collaborative Research program. *Archives of General Psychiatry, 46*(11), 971–982. doi:10.1001/archpsyc.1989.01810110013002.

Elliott, R., Bohart, A. C., Watson, J. C., & Murphy, D. (2018). Therapist empathy and client outcome: An updated meta-analysis. *Psychotherapy, 55*(4), 399–410. doi:10.1037/pst0000175.

Ellis, A. (1962). *Reason and Emotion in Psychotherapy.* Seacaucas, NJ: Citadel Press.

Eysenck, H. J. (1966). *The Effects of Psychotherapy.* New York, NY: International Science Press.

Eysenck, H. J. (1993). Forty years on: The outcome problem in psychotherapy revisited. In: T. R. Giles (Ed.), *Handbook of Effective Psychotherapy* (pp. 3–20). New York, NY: Plenum Press.

Fancher, R. T. (1995). *Cultures of Healing: Correcting the Image of American Mental Health.* New York, NY: W. H. Freeman & Co.

Fenichel, O. (1954). Symposium on the theory of the therapeutic results of psychoanalysis. In: H. Fenichel & D. Rapaport, (Eds.), *The Collected Papers of Otto Fenichel* (2nd series, pp. 19–24). New York, NY: W. W. Norton. (Work originally published 1937).

Fink, B. (1995). *The Lacanian Subject: Between Language and Jouissance.* Princeton, NJ: Princeton University Press.

Fink, B. (1997). *A Clinical Introduction to Lacanian Psychoanalysis: Theory and Technique.* Cambridge, MA: Harvard University Press.

Fink, B. (2004). *Lacan to the Letter: Reading Écrits Closely.* Minneapolis, MN: University of Minnesota Press.

94   *References*

Fink, B. (2007). *Fundamentals of Psychoanalytic Technique: A Lacanian Approach for Practitioners*. New York, NY: W. W. Norton.

Fink, B. (2014a). *Against Understanding: Commentary and Critique in a Lacanian Key (Vol 1)*. New York, NY: Routledge.

Fink, B. (2014b). *Against Understanding: Commentary and Critique in a Lacanian Key (Vol 2)*. New York, NY: Routledge.

Fink, B. (2017). *A Clinical Introduction to Freud: Techniques for Everyday Practice*. New York, NY: Norton.

Fluckiger, C., Del Re, A. C., Wampold, B. E., & Horvath, A. O. (2018). The alliance in adult psychotherapy: A meta-analytic synthesis. *Psychotherapy, 55*(4), 316–340. doi:10.1037/pst0000172.

Foucault, M. (1978). *The History of Sexuality: Vol. 1. An Introduction* (R. Hurley, Trans.). New York, NY: Vintage. (Original work published 1976).

Fowers, B. J., Richardson, F. C., & Slife, B. D. (2017). *Frailty, Suffering, and Vice: Flourishing in Face of Human Limitations*. Washington, DC: American Psychological Association.

Frank, J. D., & Frank, J. B. (1991). *Persuasion and Healing: A Comparative Study of Psychotherapy* (3rd ed.). Baltimore, MD: John Hopkins University Press.

Franklin, M. E., & Foa, E. B. (2014). Obsessive-compulsive disorder. In: D. H. Barlow (Ed.), *Clinical Handbook of Psychological Disorders: A Step-By-Step Treatment Manual* (5th ed., pp. 155–205). New York, NY: Guilford Press.

Freud, S. (1963). *Introductory Lectures on Psychoanalysis*. In: J. Strachey (Trans. & Ed.), *The* Standard Edition *of the* Complete Psychological Works *of Sigmund Freud* (Vol. 16, pp. 243–463). London: Hogarth Press. (Original work published 1917).

Freud, S. (1964). *New Introductory Lectures on Psychoanalysis*. In: J. Strachey (Trans. & Ed.), *The Standard Edition of the Complete Psychological Works of Sigmund Freud* (Vol. 22, pp. 1–182). London: Hogarth Press. (Original work published 1933).

Fromm, E. (1976). *To Have or to Be?* New York, NY: Bantam Books.

Gendlin, E. T. (1996). *Focusing-Oriented Psychotherapy: A Manual of the Experiential Method*. New York, NY: Guilford Press.

Glasofer, D. R., Albano, A. M., Simpson, H. B., & Steinglass, J. E. (2016). Overcoming fear of eating: A case study of a novel use of exposure and response prevention. *Psychotherapy, 53*(2), 223–231. doi:10.1037/pst0000048.

Gnaulati, E. (2018). *Saving Talk Therapy: How Health Insurers, Big Pharma, and Slanted Science Are Ruining Good Mental Health Care*. Boston, MA: Beacon Press.

Gray, P. (1994). *The Ego and the Analysis of Defense*. Northvale, NJ: Jason Aronson.

Greenberg, J. R., & Mitchell, S. M. (1983). *Object Relations in Psychoanalytic Theory*. Cambridge, MA: Harvard University Press.

Grencavage, L. M., & Norcross, J. C. (1990). Where are the commonalities among the therapeutic common factors? *Professional Psychology: Research and Practice, 21*(5), 372–378. doi:10.1037/0735-7028.21.5.372.

Hacking, I. (1995). The looping effects of human kinds. In: D. Sperber, D. Premack, & A. J. Premack (Eds.), *Causal Cognition: A Multidisciplinary Debate* (pp. 351–383). New York, NY: Clarendon Press/Oxford.

Hoffmann, S. G., & Barlow, D. H. (2014). Evidence-based psychological interventions and the common factors approach: The beginnings of a rapprochement? *Psychotherapy, 51*(4), 510–513. doi:10.1037/a0037045.

Horvath, A. O., Cue, B., Clark, J. M., McKay, S., Vaughn, K., & Wiseman, D. (2002). [Review of the book *The great psychotherapy debate: Models, methods and findings*, by B. Wampold]. *Psychotherapy Research, 12*(1), 108–111.

Horwitz, A. V., & Wakefield, J. C. (2007). *The Loss of Sadness: How Psychiatry Transformed Normal Sorrow into Depressive Disorder*. New York, NY: Oxford University Press.

Imber, S. D., Pilkonis, P. A., Sotsky, S. M., Elkin, I., Watkins, J. T., Collins, J. F., Shea, M. T., Leber, W. R., & Glass, D. R. (1990). Mode-specific effects among three treatments for depression. *Journal of Consulting and Clinical Psychology, 58*(3), 352–359. doi:10.1037/0022-006X.58.3.352.

Ioannidis, J. P. A. (2005). Why most published research findings are false. *PLOS Medicine, 2*(8), 696–701. doi:10.1371/journal.pmed.0020124.

Johnsen, T. J., & Friborg, O. (2015). The effects of cognitive-behavioral therapy as an anti-depressive treatment is falling: A meta-analysis. *Psychological Bulletin*. Advance online publication. doi:10.1037/bul0000015.

Kant, I. (1997). *Groundwork of the Metaphysics of Morals* (M. Gregor, Trans. & Ed.). New York, NY: Cambridge University Press. (Original Work Published 1785).

Kazdin, A. E. (2007). Mediators and mechanisms of change in psychotherapy research. *Annual Review of Clinical Psychology, 3*, 1–27. doi:10-1146/annurev.clinpsy.3.022806.091432.

Kendler, H. H. (2008). *Amoral Thoughts about Morality: The Intersection of Science, Psychology and Ethics* (2nd ed.). Springfield, IL: Charles C. Thomas.

Kernberg, O. F., Selzer, M. A., Koenigsberg, H. W., Carr, A. C., & Appelbaum, A. H. (1989). *Psychodynamic Psychotherapy of Borderline Patients*. New York, NY: Basic Books.

Keyes, C. L. M. (2007). Promoting and protecting mental health as flourishing: A complementary strategy for improving national mental health. *American Psychologist, 62*(2), 95–108. doi:10.1037/0003-066X.62.2.95.

Lambert, M. J. (2013). The efficacy and effectiveness of psychotherapy. In: M. J. Lambert (Ed.), *Handbook of Psychotherapy and Behavior Change* (6th ed., pp. 169–218). Hoboken, NJ: Wiley.

Lambert, M. J., Fidalgo, L. G., & Greaves, M. R. (2016). Effective humanistic psychotherapy processes and their outcomes. In: D. J. Cain, K. Keenan, & S. Rubin (Eds.), *Humanistic Psychotherapies: Handbook of Research and Practice* (2nd ed., pp. 49–79). Washington, DC: American Psychological Association.

Laska, K. M., Gurman, A. S., & Wampold, B. E. (2014). Expanding the lens of evidence-based practice in psychotherapy: A common factors perspective. *Psychotherapy, 51*(4), 467–481. doi:10.1037/a0034332.

Lear, J. (2003). *Therapeutic Action: An Earnest Plea for Irony*. New York, NY: Other Press.

Lear, J. (2017). *Wisdom Won from Illness: Essays in Philosophy and Psychoanalysis*. Cambridge, MA: Harvard University Press.

Levinas, E. (1969). *Totality and Infinity: An Essay on Exteriority* (A. Lingus, Trans.). Pittsburgh, PA: Duquesne University Press. (Original work published 1961).

Linehan, M. M. (1993). *Cognitive-Behavioral Treatment of Borderline Personality Disorder*. New York, NY: Guilford.

London, P. (1986). *The Modes and Morals of Psychotherapy* (2nd ed.). New York, NY: Hemisphere Publishing.

Luborsky, L., Diguer, L., Seligman, D. A., Rosenthal, R., Krause, E. D., Johnson, S., Halperin, G., Bishop, M., Berman, J. S., Schweizer, E. (1999). The researcher's own therapy allegiances: A "wild card" in comparisons of treatment efficacy. *Clinical Psychology: Science and Practice, 6*, 95–106. doi:10.1093/clipsy.6.1.95.

Luborsky, L., Singer, B., & Luborsky, L. (1975). Comparative studies of psychotherapies: Is it true that "everyone has one and all must have prizes"? *Archives of General Psychiatry, 32*(8), 995–1008. doi:10.1001/archpsyc.1975.01760260059004.

MacIntyre, A. (1985). How psychology makes itself true—Or false. In: S. Koch, & D. E. Leary (Eds.), *A Century of Psychology as a Science* (pp. 897–903). New York, NY: McGraw-Hill.

Martin, M. W. (2006). *From Morality to Mental Health: Virtue and Vice in Therapeutic Culture*. New York, NY: Oxford University Press.

Martin, D. J., Garske, J. P., & Davis, M. K. (2000). Relation of the therapeutic alliance with outcome and other variables: A meta-analytic review. *Journal of Consulting and Clinical Psychology, 68*(3), 438–450. doi:10.1037/0022-006X.68.3.438.

McGilchrist, I. (2009). *The Master and His Emissary: The Divided Brain and the Making of the Western World*. New Haven, CT: Yale University Press.

McWilliams, N. (2005). Preserving our humanity as therapists. *Psychotherapy: Theory, Research, Practice, Training, 42*(2), 139–151. doi:10.1037/0033-3204.42.2.139.

Meltzoff, J., & Kornreich, M. (1970). *Research in Psychotherapy*. New York, NY: Atherton Press.

Mill, J. S. (1979). *Utilitarianism*. Indianapolis, IN: Hackett Publishing. (Original work published 1861).

Miller, R. B. (2004). *Facing Human Suffering: Psychology and Psychotherapy as Moral Engagement*. Washington, DC: American Psychological Association.

Mitchell, S. A. (1988). *Relational Concepts in Psychoanalysis: An Integration*. Cambridge, MA: Harvard University Press.

Mitchell, S. A. (1993). *Hope and Dread in Psychoanalysis*. New York, NY: Basic Books.

Mitchell, S. A. (1997). *Influence and Autonomy in Psychoanalysis*. Hillsdale, NJ: The Analytic Press.

Mitchell, S. A. (2000). *Relationality: From Attachment to Intersubjectivity*. New York, NY: Psychology Press.

Mitchell, S. A. (2002). *Can Love Last? The Fate of Romance over Time*. New York, NY: W. W. Norton.

Mitchell, S. A., & Black, M. J. (1995). *Freud and Beyond: A History of Modern Psychoanalytic Thought*. New York, NY: Basic Books.

Munder, T., Brutsch, O., Leonhart, R., Gerger, H., & Barth, J. (2013). Researcher allegiance in psychotherapy outcome research: An overview of reviews. *Clinical Psychology Review, 33*(4), 501–511. doi:10.1016/j.cpr.2013.02.002.

Nathan, P. E., & Gorman, J. M. (1998). *A Guide to Treatments That Work*. New York, NY: Oxford University Press.

Neacsiu, A. D., & Linehan, M. M. (2014). Borderline personality disorder. In: D. H. Barlow (Ed.), *Clinical Handbook of Psychological Disorders: A Step-By-Step Treatment Manual* (pp. 394–461). New York, NY: Guilford Press.

Niles, A. N., & O'Donovan, A. (2019). Comparing anxiety and depression to obesity and smoking as predictors of major medical illnesses and somatic symptoms. *Health Psychology, 38*(2), 172–181. doi:10.1037/hea0000707.

Ogden, T. H., & Gabbard, G. O. (2010). The lure of the symptom in analytic treatment. *Journal of the American Psychoanalytic Association, 58*(3), 533–544. doi:10.1177/0003065110376080.

Open Science Collaboration. (2012). An open, large-scale, collaborative effort to estimate the reproducibility of psychological science. *Perspectives on Psychological Science, 7*(6), 657–660. doi:10.1177/1745691612462588.

Orange, D. M. (2011). *The Suffering Stranger: Hermeneutics for Everyday Clinical Practice*. New York, NY: Routledge.

Parker, G., & Fletcher, K. (2007). Treating depression with the evidence-based therapies: A critique of the evidence. *Acta Psychiatrica Scandinavica, 115*(5), 352–359. doi:10.1111/j.1600-0447.2007.01007.x.

Putnam, H. (2002). *The Collapse of the Fact/Value Dichotomy and Other Essays*. Cambridge, MA: Harvard University Press.

Richardson, F. C., Fowers, B. J., & Guignon, C. B. (1999). *Re-Envisioning Psychology: Moral Dimensions of Theory and Practice*. San Francisco, CA: Jossey-Bass.

Richardson, F. C., & Zeddies, T. J. (2004). Psychoanalysis and the good life. *Contemporary Psychoanalysis, 40*(4), 617–657.

Rieff, P. (1966). *The Triumph of the Therapeutic: Uses of Faith after Freud*. Chicago, IL: University of Chicago Press.

Robinson, D. (2010). *The Philosophy of Cognitive Behavioral Therapy: Stoic Philosophy as Rational and Cognitive Therapy*. London: Karnac Books.

Robinson, D. N. (1997). Therapy as theory and as civics. *Theory and Psychology, 7*(5), 675–681.

Rogers, C. (1951). *Client-Centered Therapy*. Boston, MA: Houghton Mifflin.

Roth, A., & Fonagy, P. (2005). *What Works for Whom?* (2nd ed.). New York, NY: Guilford.

Rowlands, M. (2012). *Can Animals Be Moral?* New York, NY: Oxford University Press.

Safran, J. D., & Muran, J. C. (2000). *Negotiating the Therapeutic Alliance: A Relational Treatment Guide*. New York, NY: Guilford Press.

Schore, A. N. (2012). *The Science of the Art of Psychotherapy.* New York, NY: W. W. Norton.

Seligman, M. E. P. (2011). *Flourish: A Visionary New Understanding of Happiness and Well-Being.* New York, NY: Free Press.

Seligman, M. E. P., & Csikszentmihalyi, M. (2000). Positive psychology: An introduction. *American Psychologist, 55*(1), 5–14. doi:10.1037//0003-066X.55.1.5.

Seligman, M. E. P., Steen, T. A., Park, N., & Peterson, C. (2005). Positive psychology progress: Empirical validation of interventions. *American Psychologist, 60*(5), 410–421. doi:10.1037/0003-066X.60.5.410.

Shedler, J. (2010). The efficacy of psychodynamic psychotherapy. *American Psychologist, 65*(2), 98–109. doi:10.1037/a0018378.

Shedler, J. (2018). Where is the evidence for "evidence-based" therapy? *Psychiatric Clinics of North America, 41*(2), 319–329. doi:10.1016/j.psc.2018.02.001.

Slife, B. D., Scott, L., & McDonald, A. (2016). The clash of theism and liberal individualism in psychotherapy: A case illustration. *Open Theology, 2*(1), 595–604. doi:10.1515/opth-2016-0047.

Smith, K. R. (2009). Psychotherapy as applied science or moral praxis: The limitations of empirically supported treatment. *Journal of Theoretical and Philosophical Psychology, 29*(1), 34–46. doi:10.1037/a0015564.

Smith, M. L., Glass, G. V., & Miller, T. I. (1980). *The Benefits of Psychotherapy.* Baltimore, MD: Johns Hopkins University Press.

Steinert, C., Munder, T., Rabung, S., Hoyer, J., & Leichsenring, F. (2017). Psychodynamic therapy: As efficacious as other empirically supported treatments? A meta-analysis testing equivalence of outcomes. *American Journal of Psychiatry, 174*(10), 943–953. doi:10.1176/appi.ajp.2017.17010057.

Stern, D. B. (1997). *Unformulated Experience: From Dissociation to Imagination in Psychoanalysis.* Hillsdale, NJ: The Analytic Press.

Stern, D. B. (2010). *Partners in Thought: Working with Unformulated Experience, Dissociation, and Enactment.* New York, NY: Routledge.

Stern, D. B. (2012). Implicit theories of technique and the values that inspire them. *Psychoanalytic Inquiry, 32*(1), 33–49. doi:10.1080/07351690.2011.553163.

Stern, D. B. (2015). *Relational Freedom: Emergent Properties of the Interpersonal Field.* New York, NY: Routledge.

Stern, D. B. (2019). *The Infinity of the Unsaid: Unformulated Experience, Language, and the Nonverbal.* New York, NY: Routledge.

Stiles, W. B. (2009). Responsiveness as an obstacle for psychotherapy outcome research: It's worse than you think. *Clinical Psychology: Science and Practice, 16*(1), 86–91. doi:10.1111/j.1468-2850.2009.01148.x.

Stiles, W. B., Honos-Webb, L., & Surko, M. (1998). Responsiveness in psychotherapy. *Clinical Psychology: Science and Practice, 5*(4), 439–458. doi:10.1111/j.1468-2850.1998.tb00166.x.

Strachey, J. (1934). The nature of the therapeutic action of psychoanalysis. *International Journal of Psycho-Analysis, 15,* 117–126.

Taylor, C. (1985a). *Human Agency and Language: Philosophical Papers (1).* Cambridge, MA: Cambridge University Press.

Taylor, C. (1985b). *Philosophy and the Human Sciences: Philosophical Papers (2).* Cambridge, MA: Cambridge University Press.

Taylor, C. (1986). Human rights: The legal culture. In: P. Ricoeur (Ed.), *Philosophical Foundations of Human Rights* (pp. 49–57). Paris: Unesco.

Taylor, C. (1989). *Sources of the Self: The Making of the Modern Identity*. Cambridge, MA: Harvard University Press.

Taylor, C. (1995b). A most peculiar institution. In: J. E. J. Altham, & R. Harrison (Eds.), *World, Mind and Ethics: Essays on the Ethical Philosophy of Bernard Williams* (pp. 132–155). New York, NY: Cambridge University Press.

Taylor, C. (2003). Ethics and ontology. *The Journal of Philosophy*, *100*(6), 305–320. doi:0022-362X/03/0006/305-20.

Taylor, C. (2007a). Modern moral rationalism. In: S. Zabala (Ed.), *Weakening Philosophy: Essays in Honour of Gianni Vattimo* (pp. 57–76). Ithaca, NY: McGill-Queen's University Press.

Taylor, C. (2007b). *A Secular age*. Cambridge, MA: Harvard University Press.

Taylor, C. (2016). *The Language Animal: The Full Shape of the Human Linguistic Capacity*. Cambridge, MA: Harvard University Press.

Thompson, M. G. (2004). *The Ethic of Honesty: The Fundamental Rule of Psychoanalysis*. New York, NY: Rodopi.

Tjeltveit, A. C. (1999). *Ethics and Values in Psychotherapy*. New York, NY: Routledge.

Tolin, D. F. (2010). Is cognitive-behavioral therapy more effective than other therapies? A meta-analytic review. *Clinical Psychology Review*, *30*(6), 710–720. doi:10.1016/j.cpr.2010.05.003.

Tolin, D. F. (2014). Beating a dead dodo bird: Looking at signal vs. noise in cognitive-behavioral therapy for anxiety disorders. *Clinical Psychology: Science and Practice*, *21*(4), 351–362. doi:10.1111/cpsp.12080.

Tolin, D. F., McKay, D., Forman, E. M., Klonsky, E. D., & Thombs, B. D. (2015). Empirically supported treatment: Recommendations for a new model. *Clinical Psychology: Science and Practice*, *22*(4), 317–338. doi:10.1111/cpsp.12122.

Wampold, B. E. (2001). *The Great Psychotherapy Debate: Models, Methods and Findings*. Mahwah, NJ: Lawrence Erlbaum.

Wampold, B. E. (2007). Psychotherapy: The humanistic (and effective) treatment. *American Psychologist*, *62*(8), 857–853. doi:10.1037/0003-066X.62.8.857.

Wampold, B. E., Fluckiger, C., Del Re, A. C., Yulish, N. E., Frost, N. D., Pace, B. T., Goldberg, S. B., Miller, S. D., Baardseth, T. P., Laska, K. M., & Hilsenroth, M. J. (2017). In pursuit of truth: A critical examination of meta-analyses of cognitive behavioral therapy. *Psychotherapy Research*, *27*(1), 14–32. doi:10.1080/105033 07.2016.1249433.

Wampold, B. E., & Imel, Z. E. (2015). *The Great Psychotherapy Debate: The Evidence for What Makes Psychotherapy Work* (2nd ed.). New York, NY: Routledge.

Wampold, B. E., Mondin, G. W., Moody, M., Stich, F., Benson, K., & Ahn, H. (1997). A meta-analysis of outcome studies comparing bona fide psychotherapies: Empirically, "All must have prizes." *Psychological Bulletin*, *122*(3), 203–215. doi:10.1037/0033.2909.122.3.203.

Webb, C. A., DeRubeis, R. J., & Barber, J. P. (2010). Therapist adherence/competence and treatment outcome: A meta-analytic review. *Journal of Consulting and Clinical Psychology*, *78*(2), 200–211. doi:10.1037/a0018912.

Westen, D., Novotny, C. M., & Thompson-Brenner, H. (2004). The empirical status of empirically supported psychotherapies: Assumptions, findings, and reporting in clinical trials. *Psychological Bulletin*, *130*(4), 631–663. doi:10.1037/0033-2909.130.4.631.

Wiggins, B. J., & Chrisopherson, C. D. (2019). The replication crisis in psychology: An overview for theoretical and philosophical psychology. *Journal of Theoretical and Philosophical Psychology*, *39*(4), 202–217. doi:10.1037/teo0000137.

Woolfolk, R. L. (1998). *The Cure of Souls: Science, Values and Psychotherapy*. San Francisco, CA: Jossey-Bass.

Woolfolk, R. L. (2015). *The Value of Psychotherapy: The Talking Cure in an Age of Clinical Science*. New York, NY: Guilford Press.

Woolfolk, R. L., & Murphy, D. (2004). Axiological foundations of psychotherapy. *Journal of Psychotherapy Integration*, *14*(2), 168–191. doi:10.1037/1053-0479. 14.2.168.

Yalom, I. D. (1980). *Existential Psychotherapy*. New York, NY: Basic Books.

Yulish, N. E., Goldberg, S. B., Frost, N. D., Abbas, M., Oleen-Junk, N. A., Kring, M., Chin, M. Y., Raines, C. R., Soma, C. S., & Wampold, B. E. (2017). The importance of problem-focused treatments: A meta-analysis of anxiety treatments. *Psychotherapy*, *54*(4), 321–338. doi:10.1037/pst0000144.

Index

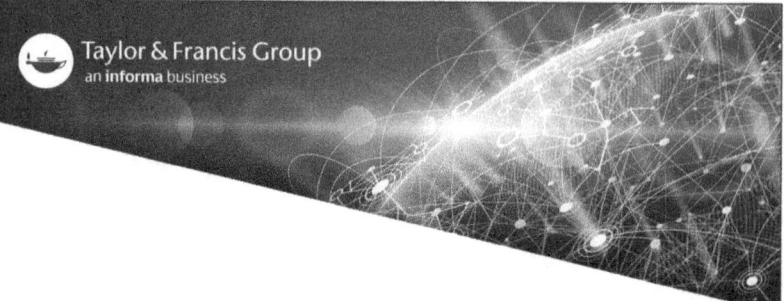
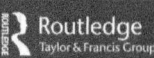
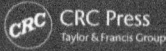